Team-Based Learning for Health Professions Education

Team-Based Learning for Health Professions Education

A Guide to Using Small Groups for Improving Learning

Edited by
Larry K. Michaelsen
Dean X. Parmelee
Kathryn K. McMahon
and
Ruth E. Levine

Foreword by Diane M. Billings

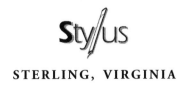

STERLING, VIRGINIA

Published by Stylus Publishing, LLC
22883 Quicksilver Drive
Sterling, Virginia 20166–2102

Library of Congress Cataloging-in-Publication Data

Team-based learning for health professions education : a guide to using small groups for improving learning / edited by Larry K. Michaelsen . . . [et al.] ; foreword by Diane M. Billings.—1st ed.

     p. ; cm.
    Includes index.
    ISBN 978–1-57922–247–5 (hardcover : alk. paper)—
    ISBN 978–1-57922–248–2 (pbk. : alk. paper)
    1. Medical education.   2. Team learning approach in education.   3. Problem-based learning.   I. Michaelsen, Larry K., 1943–
    [DNLM: 1. Education, Medical—methods.   2. Group Processes.   3. Problem-Based Learning—methods.
    W 18 T2539 2008]
    R834.T46   2008
    610.71′1—dc22   2007021701

EAN: 978–1-57922–247–5 (cloth)
EAN: 978–1-57922–248–2 (paper)

Printed in the United States of America

All first editions printed on acid free paper that meets the American National Standards Institute Z39–48 Standard.

Bulk Purchases

Quantity discounts are available for use in workshops and for staff development.
Call 1–800–232–0223

First Edition, 2008

10   9   8   7

The cover photo, by Darren Harbert, shows medical students in team-based learning at the Boonshoft School of Medicine, Wright State University.

We dedicate this book to our past, present, and future students, who deserve opportunities to learn what they need to know *and* how to use it.

We gratefully acknowledge the many faculty who have given us ideas for improving team-based learning and terrific feedback on what works and what does not. The contributors to this book have become a "team" through the months of preparation, and we thank them.

The Boonshoft School of Medicine at Wright State University provided considerable support for this project and others that have strengthened the practice of team-based learning. A special thanks for their assistance to Elizabeth Ash, Lynn Compton, and Ruth Paterson in the Office of Academic Affairs.

Contents

Foreword

Educators who facilitate learning for students in the health professions are faced with increasing challenges to promote "higher order learning," the deep and applied learning required for providing patient care in today's complex health care settings. Challenges come from varied sources including national task groups, professional organizations, institutions of higher education, and students and patients, all of whom call for relevant curricula and meaningful learning experiences to prepare graduates for safe clinical practice.

Since the Institute of Medicine published its landmark work *Crossing the Quality Chasm: A New Health System for the 21st Century* (2001), health professions educators have been challenged to respond to its recommendations for preparing a health care workforce that is able to work in teams, synthesize evidence, communicate with patients, use decision support tools, and above all else, provide safe patient care. Responding to these recommendations has required a rethinking of academic health sciences programs, often requiring the addition of content and critical synthesis skills not currently integrated into most curricula, and a revision of learning activities to include interdisciplinary teaching and learning.

The challenge of guiding student learning is made more difficult by increasing bodies of knowledge, textbooks full of rapidly outdated information, and access to Internet-based sources easily retrieved, but less easily critiqued. While "content" will continue to be the foundation of educational programs, educators now also must create opportunities for students to develop skills in acquiring, synthesizing, and using information to make clinical decisions for their patients.

There are additional challenges in the classroom. Shortages of well-prepared educators coupled with larger enrollments of increasingly diverse students demand that educators restructure their approaches to classroom learning. Generational, cultural, ethnic, gender, language, and learning style differences add another dimension that requires educators to customize educational experiences for a variety of learning needs.

It is in this context that *Team-Based Learning for Health Professions Education* arrives as a timely resource for health professions educators. This book focuses on the underlying issues of teaching and learning in the health professions—the need to engage students in active and applied learning. Early chapters in this book set the stage by explaining the premises of team-based learning, how to establish and maintain the teams, and how to create the team assignments that activate learning. The roles of the educator as learning facilitator and student as active and responsible learner are clearly delineated. Subsequent chapters give practical examples as educators from a variety of disciplines explain how to adapt and use the principles of team-based learning in their settings. Because of its tested strategies, this book undoubtedly will serve as the coach for educators as they make the long-called-for shift from teaching to learning.

Educators who use this book will transform their classrooms and find renewed satisfaction in their teaching. Students who participate in team-based learning will develop the requisite knowledge, skills, and abilities of "thinking like a professional" and face a smoother transition from student to health care provider. The patient is the ultimate beneficiary when the health practitioner has been well prepared to provide safe and effective health care.

Diane M. Billings, RN, EdD, FAAN
Chancellor's Professor Emeritus
Indiana University School of Nursing
Indianapolis, IN

Preface

The purpose of this book is to share with science and health professions educators the exciting discoveries that are being made by the application of team-based learning (TBL) to the special challenges of modern medical education.

Professors in these disciplines everywhere face three daunting challenges. First, an enormous amount of information must be learned, and it keeps growing. Second, students must learn how to use and apply that information in contexts that vary enormously between clinical cases and populations of cases. Third, in addition to these long-standing challenges, these educators, in response to public expectation, recognize the need for practitioners to have good people skills. This means learning how to communicate and collaborate effectively with coworkers, patients, and other stakeholders in the whole diagnosis/treatment/health maintenance continuum. Additionally, in many cases, instruction in the science and health professions occurs in settings of large classes, a situation not often seen as enhancing learning.

During the last decade or so, a small group of medical student educators discovered that TBL, a special way of using small-group interaction in higher education, has an extraordinary ability to effectively address all these challenges. These pioneers have been sharing their initial discoveries with each other; this book is an attempt to consolidate what has been learned in this journey and to share these ideas with an even larger number of innovators who are ready to work on improving learning in all of health and science education.

Where did the idea of TBL come from? Why is it important for teachers and others involved in health professions education to learn about it and understand it more fully?

ORIGIN OF THE IDEA OF TBL

The idea of TBL originated with Larry Michaelsen in the late 1970s. As a faculty member in the business school at the University of Oklahoma, Michaelsen was confronted with a new and daunting pedagogical challenge. Because of enrollment pressures in his department and college, he was forced to triple the size of his primary course in one semester from 40 to 120 students.

He had used group activities and assignments in the smaller classes, and this method was effective in helping students learn how to *apply* concepts, rather than simply learn *about* them. Based on this experience, he was convinced that the same kinds of group activities would work in large classes as well. As a result, he rejected the advice of his colleagues who advised turning the class into a series of lectures, in favor of an approach that involved using the vast majority of class time for group work.

By the middle of the first semester, it was obvious that this new teaching strategy was working. In fact, it was working so well that it accomplished three things that Michaelsen had not even anticipated. First, the students themselves perceived the large class setting as being far more beneficial than harmful. Second, the approach created several conditions that would enhance learning in *any* setting. In spite of the size of the class, for example, the approach was prompting most students to take responsibility for their own and their peers' learning. Third, *Michaelsen* was having fun. Because the students were getting their initial understanding of the content through their own efforts, he could concentrate his efforts on the aspect of teaching that he enjoyed most: designing assignments and activities that would enable students to discover why the subject matter that was so near and dear to him was important to them as well.

DEVELOPMENT AND REFINEMENT

After this modest but auspicious beginning, Michaelsen knew that he was on to something important, something that had major significance for other college teachers as well as for him. As a result, he has devoted much of his professional attention since that time to increasing his own understanding of why this way of using small groups works so well. He has also concentrated on helping other teachers take advantage of this innovative teaching strategy. Over time he discovered that his ability to increase his own understanding of these processes was directly related to two sets of activities.

The first set of activities relates to the research literature on the development and management of teams in multiple settings. Although he was already familiar with this literature, he was now able to read and understand it in a new way. As a result of observing hundreds of newly formed groups go through the process of maturing into effective teams, he could more clearly see the parallels between educational teams and teams in other settings. In addition, he discovered that his use of small groups raised the dynamics within groups to a new and higher level of capability. His student groups were being transformed by the TBL process into powerful learning teams, a phenomenon not well described in the literature. As a result, he was able to collect and analyze new data on the team development process and contribute articles of his own to the scholarly literature on the development and management of effective teams (Michaelsen, Watson, & Black, 1989; Watson, Kumar, & Michaelsen, 1993; Watson, Michaelsen, & Sharp, 1991).

The other activity involved making contacts with people who either used or wanted to use teams in both business and educational settings. Over the years Michaelsen has worked extensively with business executives to find ways to develop and manage effective *work* teams in corporate settings. In the academic setting, he has worked extensively to help professors find ways of building effective *learning* teams. He has conducted over 300 workshops for faculty members and published articles in a wide range of journals focused on college teaching (Michaelsen, 1983a, 1983b; 1992; 1999; Michaelsen & Black, 1994; Michaelsen, Watson, Cragin, & Fink, 1982). As a result of this involvement in both business and academia, he has both taught and been taught by thousands of people who are actively working in the trenches to develop effective teams. The most important consequence of this activity for Michaelsen is that he was able to see patterns of effective team development across a wide range of academic and business settings.

The next big step forward for TBL was when two faculty developers at Oklahoma, Dee Fink and Arletta Knight, encouraged Michaelsen to consolidate the rapidly accumulating but scattered wisdom about building the effective learning team into a more accessible form: a book and a Web site. An initial limited-edition hardback version of the book, marketed by the publisher only to libraries, was followed by a more accessible edition in paperback form: *Team-Based Learning: A Transformative Use of Small Groups in College Teaching* (Michaelsen, Knight, & Fink, 2004). Following the publication of this book, we recognized that readers and interested users would need additional resources. This led to the creation of a Web site with multiple resources to help teachers: http://www.teambasedlearning.org.

INTRODUCTION AND DEVELOPMENT IN HEALTH PROFESSIONS EDUCATION

Although a number of faculty in the health sciences had independently discovered TBL, the initial breakthrough to broader use occurred as a result of a meeting between Boyd Richards, who was on the faculty at Wake Forest, and Michaelsen's son, Doug, a second-year medical student at that institution. After an unproductive experience working in groups as they were being used there at that time, Doug approached Richards to provide some constructive criticism and to suggest an alternative—his father's ideas about in-class learning teams. Later that semester, when Michaelsen (the father) came to town to visit his son, he and Richards met for the first time and established a relationship that grew and, in time, led to a series of TBL workshops and the formation of an informal TBL faculty interest group. Unfortunately, the TBL experiment at Wake Forest stalled out because of two factors. One was that the Wake Forest faculty, both in medicine and allied health, had recently made a significant investment to adopt problem-based learning as a major component of their curricula. The other was that Richards left Wake Forest and moved to a new position at the Baylor College of Medicine.

After arriving at Baylor, Richards again invited Michaelsen to present faculty workshops on TBL. This time, however, the response was much more positive and led to a series of events that dramatically increased the visibility and potential value of TBL in health professions education. Because of increased time demands on faculty and less commitment to problem-based learning, several Baylor faculty members immediately expressed interest in the method and conducted pilot studies with favorable results. Based on the enthusiastic responses of the Baylor faculty, Richards assembled a team of interested Baylor faculty, who applied for and received one year of funding from the Fund for the Improvement of Postsecondary Education (FIPSE) to more formally evaluate the method at Baylor. After a successful year of experimentation, the team applied for and received three additional years of funding to disseminate and evaluate the method at other institutions throughout the country.

Taking advantage of their FIPSE funding, the Baylor team encouraged and supported early experimentation with the method at 10 institutions. Dean X. Parmelee and his colleagues at the Boonshoft School of Medicine at Wright State University were among the first to acquire some of the modest funding from the grant to initiate TBL at their campus, and in a two-year period were using it throughout all courses in their preclinical curriculum and in two clinical clerkships. The FIPSE support also included sponsoring an annual spring conference and providing on-site consultation. In addition, the Baylor team created assessment tools to help early adopters evaluate and disseminate the results of their experimentations, leading to publications in peer-reviewed medical education journals.

The annual conference, publications, and the ripple effect of enthusiastic users sharing their experiences with others generated interest and accelerated adoption of the method throughout the health sciences by an increasingly larger number of institutions. In fact, at the time of this writing, we would estimate that TBL is being used by at least one faculty member in 77 U.S. medical schools and at least 6 foreign countries and is being used in what is probably an even greater number of schools in other health professions programs, such as nursing, kinesiology, physician assistant, and veterinary medicine. In addition, the interest in TBL has grown into a formal organization called the Team-Based Learning Collaborative (TBLC) with an elected body of officers and a mission to promote and support TBL users in the health sciences. One of the benefits of membership in this collaborative is access to course materials (e.g., application cases) and a Listserv. As of this writing, there are 108 members in the TBLC.

REASONS FOR WRITING THIS BOOK

While Michaelsen is clearly the person who created and refined the idea of TBL, Ruth E. Levine, Kathryn K. McMahon, and Parmelee have worked closely with him for many years in writing articles and conducting workshops on TBL in medical education settings. The TBLC has held several national conferences, and its members have conducted a great many workshops and presentations on TBL at a wide range of professional organizations and health professions institutions. At the 2006 national conference at the Texas Tech Health Science Center in Lubbock, Texas, several members of the TBLC felt it was time to put pencil to paper through a book that would help more faculty to develop TBL for their courses and inspire them to contribute to the scholarship of teaching and learning in health professions education. Parmelee was recruited to lead the effort with the enthusiastic support and guidance of Levine, Michaelsen, and McMahon.

The editors and contributors to this book are convinced that TBL can truly change and transform the quality of the classroom experience for both instructor and students. They have seen their colleagues try it out and become excited about it and its potential to greatly enhance student learning. This book should help generate interest among other faculty in the various health and science professions programs and assist them with taking the next step. Many faculty and students in these programs have had small-group experiences that have been frustrating. Fortunately, the strategy of TBL addresses the core issue of accountability within small groups and proceeds to transform the small group into a real learning team. For faculty in the health professions, this book provides a terrific opportunity to learn about the effective use of small groups. We hope it will inspire readers to become more engaged with students in ways that giving lectures simply cannot do.

L. Dee Fink
Dean X. Parmelee

REFERENCES

Michaelsen, L. K. (1983a). Team learning in large classes. In C. Bouton & R. Y. Garth (Eds.), *Learning in groups* (pp. 13–22). New Directions for Teaching and Learning Series, No. 14, San Francisco: Jossey-Bass.

Michaelsen, L. K. (1983b). Developing professional competence. In C. Bouton & R. Y. Garth *(Eds.), Learning in groups* (pp. 41–57). New Directions for Teaching and Learning Series, No. 14. San Francisco: Jossey-Bass.

Michaelsen, L. K. (1992). Team-based learning: A comprehensive approach for harnessing the power of small groups in higher education. In D. H. Wulff & J. D. Nyquist (Eds.), *To improve the academy: Resources for faculty, instructional and organizational development* (Vol. 11). Stillwater, OK: New Forums Press.

Michaelsen, L. K. (1999). Myths and methods in successful small group work. *National Teaching and Learning Forum*, 8(6), 1–5.

Michaelsen, L. K., & Black, R. H. (1994). Building learning teams: The key to harnessing the power of small groups in higher education. In *Collaborative learning: A sourcebook for higher education* (Vol. 2). State College, PA: National Center for Teaching, Learning and Assessment.

Michaelsen, L. K., Knight, A. B., & Fink, L. D. (2004). *Team-based learning: A transformative use of small groups in college teaching*. Sterling, VA: Stylus.

Michaelsen, L. K., Watson, W. E., & Black, R. H. (1989). A realistic test of individual versus group consensus decision making. *Journal of Applied Psychology*, *74*(5), 834–839.

Michaelsen, L. K., Watson, W. E., Cragin, J. P., & Fink, L. D. (1982). Team-based learning: A potential solution to the problems of large classes. *Exchange: The Organizational Behavior Teaching Journal*, *7*(1), 13–22.

Watson, W. E., Kumar, K., & Michaelsen, L. K. (1993). Cultural diversity's impact on group process and performance: Comparing culturally homogeneous and culturally diverse task groups. *Academy of Management Journal*, *36*(3), 590–602.

Watson, W. E., Michaelsen, L. K., & Sharp, W. (1991). Member competence, group interaction and group decision-making: A longitudinal study. *Journal of Applied Psychology*, *76*, 801–809.

RELATED WEB SITES

General: http://www.teambasedlearning.org
Medical Education:
  1. **Baylor College of Medicine**
     http://www.bcm.tmc.edu/fac-ed/team_learning/index.html
  2. **Wright State University School of Medicine**
     http://www.med.wright.edu/aa/facdev/TBL/index.htm
  3. **The Team Learning Collaborative**
     http://www.tlcollaborative.org/
  4. **University of British Columbia**
     http://ipeer.apsc.ubc.ca/wiki/index.php/Team-Based_Learning

PART I

Fundamentals

CHAPTER 1

Team-Based Learning in Health Professions Education

Why Is It a Good Fit?

Dean X. Parmelee

CASE REPORTS FROM HEALTH PROFESSIONS EDUCATION SETTINGS

First-Year Medical Student. George is 25 years old, finished college, and worked for a couple of years as an emergency medical technician before entering medical school. He is halfway through his first year and feels overwhelmed with how much he has to memorize and regurgitate. The lectures are only occasionally good, rarely exciting, and the small-group sessions are mostly opportunities for a couple of classmates to show off what they know, and for a faculty member to give a mini lecture. Exam questions, all multiple choice, are tough because they focus on unnecessary detail, and he is experiencing a huge disconnect between all the book knowledge and what he feels he will be doing in the future as a physician.

Senior Nursing Student. Ellen, about to graduate as a nurse with a bachelor's degree, looks back upon her education and wonders if there was a better way to have learned all the science before moving into the clinicals. She almost quit several times because she was asked to solve so few meaningful problems; the emphasis was always on knowing the facts. The clinicals saved her because she had to solve real problems. She also feels that many of her classmates should have learned earlier how to work with a team; she feels it is a skill that needs practice and lots of feedback.

Professor of Anatomy at a Dental School. Dr. B has been teaching the anatomy, histology, and embryology course to dental students for 12 years. The course has been successful from the student feedback and board scores perspective, but he is tired of lecturing—only about half of the students show up, rarely do they ask questions, and he doubts that they are getting much of out of the lectures. Same thing with the small groups he and his faculty teach—the students are just not engaged and the faculty does all the work.

Veterinary Medicine Education Dean. Dean S. has had a distinguished career in science and in educating veterinarians. Her students continue to be the very best students from the sciences and truly know how to succeed in graduate school. However, she wants them to learn more about working in teams earlier and to deal with more complex clinical problems than what the usual multiple-choice exams ask.

These case reports are representative of some of the frustrations experienced by learners and instructors involved in the education of health professionals. It is the intention of this book to introduce instructors in health professions programs to team-based learning (TBL) as a way to truly engage future professionals in their education. To do so successfully, one will have to shed conceptions of the teacher-student paradigm that maintains the lecture format and focuses on covering content rather than applying knowledge.

Educators in the health professions know that students must acquire an enormous amount of information, demonstrate that they know the information by scoring well on multiple-choice exams, and then use the information in their evaluation and treatment approaches with clinical problems. So many of our curricula are designed to cover the content deemed essential for the discipline, and although curricula may have components that require the student to demonstrate integration of content elements in problem-solving exercises, it is rare that application of knowledge is the cornerstone of a curriculum's design.

Requiring graduates of professional education/training programs to demonstrate that they have the attitudes and skills to function in the health care setting is considered under the category of professional competencies, and all disciplines have defined these with outcome measures. Unfortunately, there is still a divide in which the student/trainee must first demonstrate knowledge of facts and concepts before showing any ability to integrate this information by solving problems through the exercise of judgment or clinical reasoning. And, although all health professional training programs have professional competencies for communication, interpersonal skills, and teamwork, they struggle with how to incorporate meaningful learning opportunities for these competencies and to find methods for documenting achievement.

Over 40 years ago, at McMaster University in Ontario, Canada, problem-based learning (PBL) was developed for the medical school curriculum, and many schools adopted this strategy as a way to help health care professionals develop skills working in groups to solve clinical case problems. Wide incorporation of the strategy did not occur because of the faculty resources required (each small group requires a facilitator) and, in so many settings, both students and faculty prefer to use the lecture format for classroom teaching. With a lecture format, the time commitment is not significant for the faculty, students do not have to prepare seriously, and there is no expectation for interpersonal interaction between faculty and student or student and student. PBL addressed many of the professional competencies, but the lecture format, preferred by students emerging from pre-health undergraduate programs, has held sway.

Larry Michaelsen, as professor of business at the University of Oklahoma in the late 1970s, developed a large-class strategy that dramatically changed the dynamics in the lecture hall for his course in management. At the first session, he assigned students to teams, informed them that he would not lecture and that they would learn the content of the course on their own and in teams, and that they would be applying what they learned at every class session. His role was to tell them what content they needed to master, create challenging problems for them to solve, and probe their reasoning for how they came to their conclusions. Some students felt cheated that they were not being "taught," but they quickly discovered that they were learning more in a lecture where all the students were questioning, debating, teaching one another, and even arguing!

Michaelsen spent the next several years refining the principles of TBL, as they could be applied to any subject matter that involved problem solving. For many years, he traveled to universities and colleges doing faculty development workshops on his strategy. Many who attended taught undergraduate science classes of students who were pre-health professionals and they saw TBL as a way to get them engaged in classroom problem solving. Others thought that the strategy deviated too far from traditional pedantic paradigm and that the pre-health professions students would have a hard readjustment when they went to the graduate level.

Starting in 2001, with an award by the U.S. Department of Education's Fund for the Improvement of Postsecondary Education (FIPSE) to Baylor Medical College to increase TBL in medical education, and with the publication of *Team-Based Learning: A Transformative Use of Small Groups* (Michaelsen, Knight, & Fink, 2002) and later revised and republished as *Team-Based Learning: A Transformative Use of Small Groups in College Teaching* (Michaelsen, Knight, & Fink, 2004), faculty in medical, nursing, physician assistant, dental, and veterinary schools became interested in this strategy through workshops, peer-reviewed publications, and a changing health care education environment that wanted its professionals to be better at teamwork.

Faculty at more than fifty health professions schools have tried out TBL, and there have been over 20 publications on its use with health professions education in peer-reviewed journals since the beginning of the FIPSE program. No professional degree program has adopted the strategy as the cornerstone of its curriculum, but some have used it increasingly in courses, and faculty interest continues to grow. Since so many courses in the health professions are taught by several faculty in the attempt to provide integration of science disciplines (anatomy, physiology, biochemistry), it requires one or two very determined faculty members to develop and deliver the TBL modules, sometimes stretching their comfort level with the course content. However, when several faculty from different disciplines start working together on creating TBL modules, the benefit for the students can be great, since they must integrate the content from these disciplines to be successful.

For example, an anatomist, a biochemist, and a physiologist could collaborate to develop a group application on Vitamin D. A case of rickets is selected and questions designed that require the students to demonstrate their knowledge of the anatomy and histology of bones, the formation and structure of Vitamin D, the physiology of bone formation, and how to apply this knowledge to solving complex problems on the diagnosis, treatment, and prevention of rickets. This group application then becomes the focus for a defined portion of the course's content related to normal and abnormal bone formation and structure. The faculty determines the depth of knowledge necessary to answer the group application questions, and assigns readings or other activities (histology lab, interpretation of bone density studies, question sets in biochemistry) that must be done *before* class. At the end of the exercise, the faculty will know how well the students have mastered the material and can address any important gaps in knowledge or application of the knowledge.

Clearly, this process of faculty collaboration to design and deliver an effective TBL module is more challenging and time consuming than putting the requisite lectures together to cover the content. And, the faculty must know how the student clinicians (dental, medical students) solve problems at their stage of education so that they can tailor the difficulty and complexity of the questions. Students in a program designed to produce research scientists will need to have not only very complex questions, but also ones that require considerable creativity to answer and defend. Faculty hesitation to incorporate TBL in a course, or convert the course to TBL, is understandable, but we feel that for professional students to be engaged fully, challenged intellectually, and have the opportunity to develop interpersonal and teamwork skills, the TBL strategy holds the greatest promise in curriculum development.

Student engagement is the hallmark of TBL. As experienced educators know, student engagement with content is correlated with both student satisfaction and student achievement, especially when the subject matter is difficult. The well-designed TBL module, used in a class where teams have been properly created, generates remarkable interactions between students and the faculty instructor. There is no comparison between what one sees and hears in such a class and a lecture format class. Furthermore, the longer teams work together with appropriately challenging TBL modules, the more they appreciate being given progressively difficult problems to solve.

What is it about the TBL strategy that guarantees student engagement? It is all about accountability and learning about judgment.

Accountability

It is part of the structure of TBL. Students learn quickly that their grades as individuals in the course are derived from how well they prepare for TBL sessions (individual Readiness Assurance Test), how well they relate to their team members and contribute to their team's productivity (peer evaluation), how well they as team members can demonstrate their collective preparation (group Readiness Assurance Test), and how well they collaborate as team members to apply their knowledge to solve difficult problems (group application exercise). Although all of these grade incentives for accountability motivate the students to work hard, they become less important as teams work together over time. Members of established learning teams report that they prepare thoroughly and contribute all they can in the sessions because they want their team to be successful. The lecture format can never generate the level of engagement with content that comes from students using their cognition and their affect through the TBL process.

Judgment

Kenneth A. Bruffee (1978), defined judgment as "decision making, discrimination, evaluation, analysis, synthesis, establishing or recognizing conceptual frames of reference, and defining facts within them" (p. 450).

Health professionals become clinicians when they are given responsibility to care for others. In addition to a host of personal characteristics, such as a passion to provide service to others, the clinician must have this judgment skill set to make decisions. The structure of TBL requires the individual and the team to judge and make decisions, and when the instructor facilitates well, both individuals and teams must explain how they arrived at their decisions and why they excluded other considerations. The entire process of dialogue and debate within teams and between teams teaches students about judgment, and, as they practice the skill set for judgment, they engage deeply with the content. Many of us would consider judgment to be the foundation of sound clinical reasoning.

As one reads the remaining chapters of this book, one will discover that TBL holds much promise to transform the way health professions education and its related science disciplines are taught and learned. The strategy's inherent approach to accountability, judgment, and the mastery of content for the purpose of applying it in the classroom supports the values and competencies that prepare the student for a future as a professional. Furthermore:

- It is suitable for large classes held in lecture halls.
- It engages students fully during class time.
- Students come to class on time and they come prepared.
- One faculty member can conduct an entire session.
- Several professional competencies can be addressed (communication, interpersonal skills, teamwork skills, including giving and receiving peer feedback, knowledge acquisition, and applying knowledge to real case problems).
- Academic achievement on end-of-course exams is the same or better than with traditional lecture format.
- It offers students opportunities to develop clinical reasoning skills in the context of a supportive and engaged group of peers.
- It contributes to the development of a learning community for a class.

The chapters that follow in this book intend to prepare instructors in the health professions to create and deliver TBL sessions. The next two chapters by Michaelsen and Sweet provide details on the structure and process of TBL so that one can envision how to do it and try it out. Other chapters give additional hands-on approaches to selecting teams and enhancing their productivity, and how to use peer evaluation. Because of the burgeoning interest in understanding better how future clinicians develop their clinical reasoning, chapter 4 reviews critical thinking in the context of TBL.

For a relatively new educational strategy to grow in acceptance and use, its outcomes must be published in the peer-reviewed literature; therefore, in chapter 10 three scholars have written about what they feel are the scholarship priorities for TBL. Part two, "Voices of Experience," is by contributors who have taken the plunge and started using TBL in their classes. Not always have they followed the rules for how to do it; sometimes, they have discovered some variations that work well in their particular setting.

Several faculty at my institution, the Boonshoft School of Medicine at Wright State University, began to use TBL in our preclinical curriculum in 2002. Within one year, all of our preclinical, basic medical science courses were incorporating TBL as important components of the course work. Over the next four years, faculty learned more about how to do it well, and we created a culture that supported it. Student evaluations of TBL have become uniformly excellent and faculty who use it would never go back to the previous small-group teaching. We continue to expand its use in our curriculum and to learn how to generate the best learning for our students.

REFERENCES

Bruffee, K. A. (1978). The Brooklyn plan: Attaining intellectual growth through peer group tutoring. *Liberal Education, 64*(4), 447–468.

Michaelsen, L. K., Knight, A. B., & Fink, L. D. (Eds.). (2002). *Team-based learning: A transformative use of small groups.* Westport, CT: Praeger.

Michaelsen, L. K., Knight, A. B., & Fink, L. D. (Eds.). (2004). *Team-based learning: A transformative use of small groups in college teaching.* Sterling, VA: Stylus.

Chapter 2

Fundamental Principles and Practices of Team-Based Learning

Larry K. Michaelsen and Michael Sweet

Team-based learning (TBL) differs from other forms of small-group work in that it involves developing and using learning teams as an instructional *strategy*. As a result, implementing TBL typically requires linking each learning activity to the next and explicitly designing assignments to accomplish two purposes: deepening students' learning and promoting the development of high-performance learning teams.

We are all familiar with the look and feel of traditional, lecture-based instruction—as students, we learned that lecturing is what college teaching was mostly about—and many of us carried that model of teaching into our own early careers as professors. When coming from a chalk-'n-talk background, implementing TBL requires a fundamental change in the way you think about what happens in classrooms and laboratories. Traditionally, teachers have focused on *teaching* with an emphasis on facts and ideas and how best to present them. In contrast, the TBL instructor focuses on *learning*, and the emphasis is on what the students are *doing* in the classroom and how they are learning from their experience.

The goal of this chapter is to describe the key characteristics of TBL and how it can best be implemented as an instructional strategy. Throughout, we will emphasize that the tremendous power of TBL is derived from a single factor: the high level of cohesiveness and trust that can be developed within student learning groups while never stepping away from course content. In other words, the effectiveness of TBL as an instructional strategy is based on the fact that it *nurtures the development of high levels of group cohesiveness and trust among students as a natural result of* how *content is covered in class*. In TBL, the cohesiveness and trust that develops among team members derives from the *sequence* and *structure* of content-mastery activities. As the course unfolds, this cohesiveness development makes possible increasingly rich and motivated discussion among students, generating a wide variety of other positive outcomes. When one fully understands the importance of group cohesiveness and trust as the foundation for powerful learning teams, the significance of the procedures described in this chapter become clear.

The development of a small group into a learning team is best described as a *transformation process* (see chapter 4 in Michaelsen, Knight, & Fink, 2002, 2004).

The paragraphs that follow will outline a set of principles and practices that are critical to this transformation process. Part one of this chapter presents *four essential principles* for implementing TBL, part two provides a discussion of the steps involved in actually implementing TBL, and part three briefly outlines some of the primary benefits of using TBL.

PART ONE—FOUR ESSENTIAL PRINCIPLES OF TBL

Shifting from traditional forms of teaching to a TBL approach requires significant changes in (a) the focus of the *learning objectives* for a given course, (b) the nature of the *classroom events* intended to achieve these objectives, and (c) the *role* played by the instructor and students within these events.

The primary learning objective of most classes is to familiarize students with course concepts. By contrast, the primary learning objective in TBL (and one that is completely consistent with the demands of health professions education) is to ensure that students have the opportunity to practice *using course concepts to solve problems*. Thus with TBL, although some time is spent on ensuring that students master the course content, the vast majority of class time is used for team assignments that focus on *using* course content to solve the kinds of problems that students are likely to face as practicing professionals. This, in turn, requires that the instructor's primary role shift from dispensing information to designing and managing the overall instructional process. Furthermore, instead of being passive recipients of information, students are required to accept responsibility for the initial exposure to the course content so that they will be prepared for the in-class teamwork. Changes of this magnitude do not happen automatically. They are, however, reliable and natural outcomes when the four essential principles of TBL have been implemented.

The four essential principles of TBL are:

1. Groups must be properly formed *and* managed.
2. Students must be accountable for the quality of their individual *and* group work.
3. Students must have frequent *and* timely feedback.
4. Team assignments must promote both learning *and* team development.

When courses are designed and managed so that these principles are implemented, student groups naturally evolve into cohesive learning teams.

Principle 1—Groups Must Be Properly Formed *and* Managed

Forming effective groups requires that the instructor oversee the formation of the groups so that he or she can manage three important variables. One is ensuring that the groups have adequate and approximately the same level of resources to draw from in completing their assignments. The second is ensuring that the groups have the opportunity to develop into learning teams. The third is avoiding establishing groups whose membership characteristics are likely to interfere with the development of group cohesiveness.

Distributing Member Resources

In order for groups to function as effectively as possible, they should also be as diverse as possible. That is, every group needs access to the students who have the potential for making a significant contribution to the success of their group. Thus, each group should contain a mix of student characteristics in relation to the course content (e.g., previous course work and/or course-related practical experience) as well as demographic characteristics like gender, ethnicity, and so on. Further, teams will develop faster when relevant member characteristics are evenly distributed across the groups. However, students intuitively have neither enough information nor the inclination to wisely form groups; therefore the task must always be the responsibility of the instructor. (For specific methods for grouping students see http://www.team basedlearning.org; Michaelsen et al., 2002, pp. 40–41; 2004, pp. 39–40; and chapter 6 and Appendix 2.A in this book.) Because TBL assignments involve highly challenging intellectual tasks, teams must be fairly large and diverse. Specifically, we recommend that teams should be composed of five to seven members and be as heterogeneous as possible. If teams are smaller and/or homogeneous, some are likely to face the problem of not having a sufficiently rich talent pool of individual resources needed to be successful—especially on days when one or more team members are not present in the class (see chapter 4 in Michaelsen et al., 2002, 2004).

Time—A Key Factor in Team Development

Students should stay in the same group for the entire course. Although even a single well-designed group assignment usually produces a variety of positive outcomes, only when students work together over time can their groups become cohesive enough to evolve into self-managed and truly effective learning teams (see chapter 4 in Michaelsen et al., 2002, 2004; and chapter 6 and Appendix 2.A in this book). Team development occurs through a series of interactions that enable individual members to test the extent to which they can trust their peers to take them seriously and treat them fairly. Newly formed groups tend to rely heavily on their one or two most assertive (although not always most competent) members and have not yet learned how and when to tap into the resources that reside throughout the group. Under the right conditions, however, the vast majority of groups learn how to interact much more productively. In addition, although member diversity initially inhibits group processes and performance, it eventually becomes a clear asset when members have worked together over an extended period of time (Watson, Kumar, & Michaelsen, 1993).

As groups develop into teams, communication becomes more open and far more conducive to learning. In part, this occurs because trust and understanding build to the point where members are willing and able to engage in intense give-and-take interactions without having to worry about being offensive or misunderstood. In addition (and in contrast to temporary groups), members of mature teams become more willing to challenge each other because they see their own success as being integrally tied to the success of their team. Thus, over time, members' initial concerns about creating a bad impression by being "wrong" are outweighed by their motivation to ensure the success of their team (see chapter 4 in Michaelsen et al., 2002, 2004). When this occurs, studies have shown that 98% of teams will outperform their own best member on learning-related tasks (Michaelsen, Watson, & Black, 1989).

Minimizing Barriers to Group Cohesiveness—Avoiding Coalitions

The greatest threats to group cohesiveness development are coalitions: either a previously established relationship between a subset of members in the group (e.g., boyfriend/girlfriend, fraternity brothers, etc.) or the potential for a cohesive subgroup based on background factors such as nationality, culture, or native language. In newly formed groups, these factors are likely to become the basis for insider/outsider tension, which can plague the group for the entirety of a course. As a result, allowing students to form their own groups practically ensures the existence of potentially disruptive subgroups and must be avoided (Fiechtner & Davis, 1985; Michaelsen & Black, 1994). Thus, teachers should use a group formation process that mixes students up in a way that forces all groups to build into teams from the ground up. (For specific methods for grouping students see Michaelsen et al., 2002, pp. 40–41; 2004, pp. 39–40; http://www.teambasedlearning.org; and chapters 2 and 6 of this book).

Principle 2—Students Must Be Accountable for the Quality of Their Individual *and* Group Work

In traditional classes, there is no real need for students to be accountable to anyone other than the instructor. Thus, it is possible to establish a sufficient degree of accountability by simply assigning grades to students' work. By contrast, with TBL it is essential for individual students to be accountable to both the instructor and their team for the quality and quantity of their individual work. Further, teams must also be accountable for the quality and quantity of their work as a unit.

Establishing this accountability requires creating two conditions. One is ensuring that the quality of students' individual and teamwork can be monitored. The other is ensuring that the quality of their work will have consequences (good and bad) that are significant enough to motivate high-quality work. The paragraphs below describe how the various practices that are part of TBL promote accountability for the behaviors that are critical to successful teamwork and individual learning.

Accountability for Individual Preclass Preparation

Lack of preparation places clear limits on individual learning and team development. If several members of a team come unprepared to contribute to a complex group task, then the team as a whole is far less likely to succeed at that task, cheating its members of the learning the task was designed to stimulate. No amount of discussion can overcome absolute ignorance. Furthermore, lack of preparation also hinders cohesiveness development because those who do make the effort to be prepared will resent having to carry their peers. As a result, the effective use of learning groups clearly requires individual students to be made accountable for class preparation.

In TBL, the basic mechanism that ensures individual accountability for preclass preparation is the Readiness Assurance Process (RAP) that occurs at the *beginning* of each major unit of instruction (see below and in Michaelsen & Black, 1994). The first step in the process is an individual Readiness Assurance Test (RAT; typically 10–20 multiple-choice questions) over a set of preclass assignments, for example, readings, lab exercises, dissections, etc. Students then turn in their individual answers and are given an additional answer sheet to retake the same test as a team, coming to a consensus on their team answers. This process promotes students' accountability to the instructor and to each other. First, students are responsible to the instructor because the individual scores count as part of the course grade (discussed in detail below). Second, during the group test, each member is invariably asked to voice and defend his or her choice on every question. As a result, students are clearly and explicitly accountable to their peers for not only completing their preclass assignments, but also for being able to explain the concepts to each other.

Accountability for Contributing to Their Team

The next step is ensuring that members contribute time and effort to group work. In order to accurately assess members' contributions to the success of their teams, it is imperative that instructors involve the students themselves in a peer assessment process. That is, members should be given the opportunity to evaluate one another's contributions to the activities of the team. Contributions to the team include individual preparation for teamwork, reliable class attendance, attendance at team meetings that may occur outside of class, positive contributions to team discussions, valuing and encouraging input from fellow team members, and so on. Peer assessment is essential because team members are typically the only ones who have enough information to accurately assess one another's contributions. (See chapter 9 and part two in this book for additional information on peer evaluations.)

Accountability for High-Quality Team Performance

The third significant factor in ensuring accountability is developing an effective means to assess team performance. There are two keys to effectively assessing teams. One is using assignments that require teams to create a product that can be readily compared across teams and with expert opinions (including those of the instructor— see below). The other is using procedures to ensure that such comparisons occur frequently and in a timely manner (see below).

Principle 3—Students Must Receive Frequent *and* Timely Feedback

Immediate feedback is the instructional prime mover in TBL for two very different reasons. First, feedback is *essential* to content learning and retention—a notion that not only makes intuitive sense but is also well documented in educational research literature (e.g., Bruning, Schraw, & Ronning, 1994). The second reason immediate feedback is crucial to TBL is seldom mentioned in the education literature but *is* well documented in decades of group dynamics research (see chapter 4 in Michaelsen et al., 2002, 2004)—feedback is important because of its impact on team development. Further, the positive impact of feedback on learning and team development is greater when it is immediate, frequent, and discriminatory (i.e., enables learners to clearly distinguish between good and bad choices, effective and ineffective strategies, etc.).

Timely Feedback From the RATs

The RATs—mentioned above and discussed in detail later in this chapter—are where TBL provides students the feedback they need for learning and team development. Since RATs are given at the beginning of each major instructional unit, they virtually guarantee that students will have the conceptual skills required for tackling more complex application-focused assignments. In addition, feedback from the group RATs facilitates team development in two important ways. One is that because the group (not individual) scores are made public, members are highly motivated to pull together to protect their public image. The other is that immediate feedback during the group tests stimulates groups to continually improve how they communicate as a team. Because they receive the real-time feedback during the team test, students can instantly reflect on how their group failed to capitalize on the knowledge of one or more of their members—strongly motivating them to keep it from happening next time (Watson, Michaelsen, & Sharp, 1991). Thus, over time, naturally extroverted or assertive members learn to do more listening and less talking, quieter students become much more active in team discussions, and cohesiveness increases because members develop a genuine appreciation for each other's contributions.

Timely Feedback on Application-Focused Team Assignments

Providing immediate feedback on application-focused team assignments is just as important for learning and team development, but this typically presents a much greater challenge than providing immediate feedback on the RATs. Unlike the RATs, which are designed to ensure that students understand basic concepts, most application-focused team assignments are aimed at developing higher-level thinking skills in more complex situations. As a result, these assignments can be much more difficult to design and grade, but the task is fairly straightforward once you understand the key elements in the process (see chapter 3).

In fact, many assignments you already use can likely be modified to facilitate learning and team development as TBL application-oriented activities. For example, one instructor already used a series of case write-ups to develop her medical students' diagnostic skills. She used to require student groups to write a series of one-page memos identifying a preliminary diagnosis of the patients in each case. Unfortunately, groups almost always simply divided the cases across their members, which resulted in students actively working with (and learning from) only a fraction of the cases. Furthermore, because of the large class size, she had to spend considerable time reading responses for the grading.

When she started using TBL, she modified these assignments in two ways. First, she placed the emphasis on *deciding* on a diagnosis rather than writing about it. Second, she involved the teams in the assessment/feedback process. Now, she preassigns the same set of cases—all students must read the cases outside class and come prepared to help develop a diagnosis for each case. In class, however, the teacher adds a vital piece of new information to the assigned case and gives teams a specified length of time to either (a) select a most likely diagnosis from a limited set of alternatives, or (b) commit to a position that one simply cannot make a definite diagnosis with the information provided. When the time for deciding has elapsed, the teams hand in a one-page form on which they report their choice and the key items of evidence supporting their conclusion (for grading purposes). Once teams have turned in their decisions, she asks the teams to simultaneously hold up a numbered card revealing their diagnostic choice and then walks through the case with the whole class by having the teams defend their choice. In this form, the outcome of each case assignment is a *series* of lively discussions. The discussions first occur *within* the teams. Then, there is always a vigorous interchange *between* all teams, as students challenge the rationale for each other's choices. Further, the give-and-take discussions in both phases fosters concept understanding *and* team cohesiveness.

Principle Four—Team Assignments Must Promote Both Learning *and* Team Development

The development of *appropriate* group assignments is a critical aspect of successfully implementing TBL. In fact, most of the reported problems with learning groups (free riders, member conflict, etc.) are the direct result of inappropriate group assignments. When bad assignments are used, poor results are predictable and very nearly 100% preventable. In most cases, the reason that group assignments produce problems is that they are not really group assignments at all. Instead, the structure of the assignment is such that individuals working alone rather than members working together as a group wind up doing the actual work. Further, since discussion time is so limited, these kinds of assignments inhibit learning and *prevent*, rather than promote, team development.

The most fundamental aspect of designing effective team assignments is ensuring that they truly require group interaction. In most cases, team assignments will generate a high level of interaction if they (a) require teams to use course concepts to make *decisions* that involve a complex set of issues, and (b) enable teams to report their decisions in a simple form. When assignments emphasize making decisions, intragroup discussion is the natural and rational way to complete the task. In contrast, assignments that involve producing complex outputs, such as a lengthy document, are likely to limit discussion because the rational way to complete the task is to divide up the work and have members individually complete their part of the total task. Therefore, tasks that can be divided among team members should always be avoided. (A thorough discussion of effective team assignments follows in chapter 3).

Conclusion

By adhering to the four essential principles of TBL, teachers ensure that the vast majority of groups will develop a level of cohesiveness and trust required to transform them into effective learning teams. Appropriately forming the teams puts them on equal footing and greatly reduces the possibility of mistrust from preexisting relationships between a subset of team members. Holding students accountable for preparing for and attending class motivates team members to behave in ways that build cohesiveness and foster trust. Using RATs and other assignments to provide ongoing and timely feedback on individual and team performance enables teams to develop confidence in their ability to capture the intellectual resources of all their members. Assignments that promote learning and team development motivate members to challenge each other's ideas for the good of the team. Also, over time students' confidence in their teams grows to the point where they are willing and able to tackle difficult assignments with little or no external help.

PART TWO—IMPLEMENTING TBL

Effectively using TBL typically requires redesigning a course from beginning to end, and the redesign process should begin well before the start of the school term. The redesign process involves making decisions about and/or designing activities at four different points in time. These are (a) before class begins, (b) the first day of class, (c) each major unit of instruction, and (d) near the end of the course.

Before Class Begins

As described in chapter 1, traditional health professions education starts with a lengthy knowledge-acquisition/knowledge-application phase that spans several academic terms or even years. During that time, students take a series of lecture-based courses in which they are asked to absorb a great deal of knowledge that they will then later (sometimes much later) be asked to put to use.

TBL, however, uses a fundamentally different knowledge-acquisition/knowledge-application model. With TBL, students repeat the knowledge-acquisition/

knowledge-application cycle several times *within each individual course*. With TBL, students individually study the course content, discuss it with their peers and the instructor (see the RAP below) and immediately apply it in solving problems much like those they will face in professional practice. Thus, students in TBL courses develop a much better sense of the relevance of the material because they seldom have to make inferences about when and how the content might become useful in the real world. Rather than being filled with libraries of "inert knowledge" (Whitehead, 1929) from which they then later must extract needed information with great effort, students walk away from TBL courses having already begun the practical, problem-solving process of learning to use their knowledge in context.

This benefit, however, does not occur by accident. Designing a successful TBL course involves making decisions related to (a) identifying the instructional goals and objectives, (b) partitioning the course content into macro units and identifying the key concepts for each unit, and (c) designing a grading system for the course.

Backward Design

Designing a TBL course requires instructors to think backward to deal effectively with care design decisions. What do we mean by *think backward*? In most forms of higher education, teachers traditionally design their courses by asking themselves what they feel students need to *know*, then telling the students that information, and finally testing the students on how well they absorbed what they were told. In TBL, courses are not organized initially around what you want the students to *know*, but instead what you want them to be able to *do*. Wiggins and McTighe (1998) coined the term "backwards design" to describe the process of building courses this way, and its benefits are intuitively obvious: as any experienced doctor will tell you, being able to recite all the subtle differences between one form of a disease and another is a very different kind of knowledge than being able to quickly diagnose the correct form of that disease suffered by a real, living patient.

What are students who really "get it" *doing*? Imagine you are working shoulder to shoulder with students from not so long ago, and in a wonderful moment you see them do something that makes you think, "Hooray! They *really* got from my class what I *wanted* them to get—*there's the evidence!*"

When designing a course backward, the question you ask yourself is: *What, specifically, is that evidence?* What could students be doing in that wonderful moment to make it obvious they really internalized what you were trying to teach them and are putting it to use in the world?

For every course there are several answers to this question, and these different answers will correspond to the macro units of the redesigned version of the course. A given real-world moment will likely demand knowledge from one part of a course but not another. So for any given course, you should brainstorm about a half dozen of these proud moments in which a former student is making it obvious that he or she really learned what you wanted the student to learn. For now, don't think about

the classroom, just imagine the student is doing something in a real clinical or laboratory context. Also, don't be afraid to get too detailed as you visualize these
moments—in fact come up with as many details as you can about *how* this former
student is doing what he or she is doing, what *decisions* the student is making, in
what *sequence*, under what *conditions*, and so on.

These detailed scenarios become useful in three ways. First, the actions taking
place in the scenarios will help you organize your course into macro units. Second,
the scenarios will enable you to use your class time to build students' applied knowledge instead of inert knowledge. Third, the details of the scenario will help you
design the criteria for the assessments upon which you can base your students' grades.

Once you have brainstormed your "Aha! They got it!" scenarios and the details
that accompany them, let's step into the classroom. Those half dozen or so scenarios
are what you want your students to be able to *do* when they have completed your
class: they are your instructional objectives. Now you are ready to ask three more
questions:

1. **What will students need to *know* in order to be able to *do* those things?**
   Answers to this question will guide your selection of a textbook, the contents of
   your course packet, laboratory exercises, and will likely prompt you to provide
   supplementary materials of your own creation or, simply, reading guides to help
   students focus on what you consider most important in the readings or lab findings. In addition, it will be key in developing questions for the RATs (see below).

2. **While solving problems, what knowledge will students need to make
   decisions?**
   Answers to this question will help you import the use of course knowledge from
   your brainstormed real-world scenarios into the classroom. You may not be able
   to bring the actual clinical or laboratory settings in which your scenarios occurred
   into the classroom (although digital video, simulation mannequins, computer
   animations, and so on are coming much closer to approaching "real"), but you
   can provide enough relevant information about those settings to design activities
   that require your students to face the same kinds of problems and to make the
   same kinds of decisions they will make in the clinical and laboratory settings.

3. **What *criteria* separate a well-made decision from a poorly made decision
   using this knowledge?**
   Answers to this question will help you begin building the measures you will use
   to determine how well the students have learned the material *and* how well they
   can put it to use under specific conditions.

In summary, TBL leverages the power of action-based instructional objectives to
not only expose students to course content but also give them practice using it. When
determining an instructional objective, it is crucial to know how you are going to
assess the extent to which students have mastered that objective. Some teachers feel
that designing assessments first removes something from the value of instruction—
that it simply becomes "teaching to the test." Our view is that yes, you absolutely

should teach to the test, as long as the test represents (as closely as possible) the real use students will ultimately apply the course material to: what they are going to do with it, not just what they should know about it.

Designing a Grading System

The third step in redesigning the course is to ensure that the grading system is designed to reward the right things. An effective grading system for TBL must (a) provide incentives for individual contributions and effective work by the teams, as well as (b) address the equity concerns that naturally arise when group work is part of an individual's grade. The primary concern here is typically borne from past group work situations in which students were saddled with free-riding team members and have resented it ever since. Students worry that they will be forced to choose between getting a low grade or carrying their less-motivated peers. Instructors worry that they will have to choose between grading rigorously and grading fairly.

Fortunately, all of the above concerns are alleviated by a grading system in which a significant proportion of the grade is based on (a) individual performance, (b) team performance, and (c) each member's contributions to the success of their teams. As long as that standard is met, the primary remaining concern is that the relative weight of the factors is acceptable to both the instructor and the students. (Assigning relative weight is addressed in the next section.)

The First Hours of Class: Getting Started on the Right Foot

Activities that occur during the first few hours of class are critical to the success of TBL. During that time, the teacher must see that four objectives are accomplished. The first objective is ensure that students understand *why* you (the instructor and/or course director) has decided to use TBL and what that means about the way the class will be conducted. The second objective is to actually form the groups. The third and fourth objectives include alleviating students' concerns about the grading system and setting up mechanisms to encourage the development of positive group norms.

Introducing Students to TBL

Because TBL is so fundamentally different from traditional instructional practice, it is absolutely critical that students understand both the rationale for using TBL and what that means about the way the class will be conducted. Educating the students about TBL requires (at a minimum) providing students with an overview of the basic features of TBL, how TBL affects the role of the instructor and their role as students and why they are likely to benefit from their experience in the course. This information should be printed in the course syllabus, presented orally by the instructor, and demonstrated by one or more activities.

In order to foster students' understanding of TBL, we typically use two activities. The first involves explaining the basic features of TBL using overhead transparencies (or a PowerPoint presentation) including a discussion of the way in which learning objectives for this course will be accomplished through the use of TBL, as compared to a course that is taught with a more traditional approach. (see Appendix D-A1.1 and D-A1.2 in Michaelsen et al., 2002, 2004). The second activity, which, with class periods of less than an hour, might occur on day two, involves using part of the first class as a demonstration of a RAT (see below) using either the course syllabus or a short reading on TBL and/or about giving helpful feedback (see Michaelsen & Schultheiss, 1988) as the content material to be covered.

Forming the Groups

As discussed above, two factors must be taken into consideration when forming the groups: (a) the course-relevant characteristics of the students, and (b) the potential for the emergence of subgroups. As a result, the starting point in the group formation process is to gather information about specific student characteristics that will make it easier or more difficult for a student to succeed in *this* class. For a particular course, characteristics that could make it easier for a student to succeed might include such things as previous relevant course work or practical experience, access to perspectives from other cultures, and so on. Most commonly, student characteristics making it more difficult for them to succeed are the absence of those that would make it easier, but might include such things as a lack of language fluency.

The second factor that can affect student performance in a group is the presence of built-in subgroups, for example, boy/girl friends, sorority/fraternity members, ethnic groups, and so forth. Regardless of the process used to form the groups, both of these categories of individual member *characteristics* need to be *evenly distributed* across the groups (for specific methods for grouping students see Michaelsen et al., 2002, pp. 40–41; 2004, pp. 39–40; http://www.teambasedlearning.org; and chapter 6 in this book).

We recommend actually forming the groups in class in the presence of the students as a means of avoiding student concerns about ulterior motives the instructor may have had in forming groups. We begin the group formation process by simply asking questions about the factors that are important to group success. For a class in pharmacology, typical questions could include, "How many of you have worked as a pharmacist?" "How many have completed more than one class in biochemistry?" "How many of you attended high school outside of the United States?" and so forth. Students respond to each of the questions either orally or with a show of hands. Then, we create a stratified sampling frame by having students possessing a series of specific assets form a single line around the perimeter of the classroom with the rarest and/or most important category at the front of the line. After students are lined up, we have them count off down the line by the total number of groups (five to seven members) in the class. All "ones" become Group 1, all "twos" become Group 2, and so on. Following this procedure rapidly creates heterogeneous (and approximately equivalent-ability) teams (see Appendix 2.A).

Alleviating Student Concerns About Grades

The next step in getting started on the right foot with TBL is to address student concerns about the grading system. Fortunately, student anxiety based on previous experience largely evaporates as students come to understand two of the essential features of TBL. One is that two elements of the grading system create a high level of individual accountability for preclass preparation and class attendance—counting individual scores on the RATs and basing part of the grade on a peer evaluation. The other reassuring feature is that team assignments will be done *in class* and will be based on thinking, discussing, and deciding, so it is highly unlikely that one or two less-motivated teammates members can put the group at risk.

Years of experience have taught us that the most effective way to alleviate student concerns about grades is to directly involve students in customizing the grading system to *this* class. Students become involved by participating in an exercise called Setting Grade Weights (Michaelsen, Cragin, & Watson, 1981; Appendix B in Michaelsen et al., 2002, 2004). Within limits set by the instructor, representatives of the newly formed teams negotiate with one another to reach consensus (i.e., all of the representatives must agree) on a mutually acceptable set of weights for each of the grade components: individual performance, team performance, and members' contributions to the success of their teams. After an agreement has been reached regarding the grade weight for each component, the standard applies for all groups for the remainder of the course.

Using Each Major Unit of Instruction

Units of instruction in TBL (each consisting of approximately 6–10 class hours) follow the activity sequence shown in Figure 2.1. As described in part one, each in-class activity should be designed to build students' understanding of course content and increase group cohesiveness via proper design and immediate feedback.

FIGURE 2.1
Team-Based Learning Instructional Activity Sequence

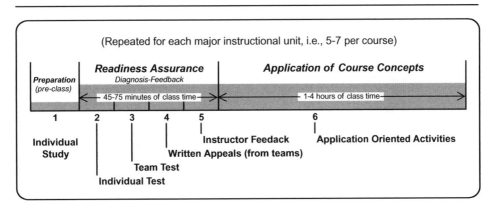

Ensuring Content Coverage

In TBL, the basic mechanism to ensure that students are exposed to course content is the Readiness Assurance Process (RAP). This process occurs five to seven times per course and constitutes the *first* set of in-class activities for each of the major instructional units identified through the backward design activity (see above). It also provides the foundation for individual and team accountability as one of the building blocks of TBL (see above). The RAP has five major components: (a) assigned readings, (b) individual tests, (c) group tests, (d) an appeals process, and (e) instructor feedback (see Table 2.1). Each of the individual components is discussed in the following paragraphs.

Assigned Readings

Prior to the beginning of each major instructional unit, students are given reading and other assignments that should contain information on the concepts and ideas that must be understood to be able to solve the problem the instructor identified for this unit in the backward design activity (see above). Students are to complete the assignments and come to the next class period prepared to take a test on the assigned materials.

**TABLE 2.1
Readiness Assurance Process**

1. Assigned Readings. In most instances, students are initially exposed to concepts through assigned readings.
2. Individual Test. Additional exposure during the individual test helps reinforce students' memory of what they learned during their individual study (for a discussion of the positive effects of testing on retention see Nungester & Duchastel, 1982).
3. Team Test. During team tests students orally elaborate the reasons for their individual answer choices. As a result, they are exposed to peer input that aids in strengthening and/or modifying their schemata related to the key course concepts. In addition, they gain from acting in a teaching role (for a discussion of the cognitive benefits of teaching see Bargh & Schul, 1980; Slavin & Karweit, 1981).
4. Appeals. During this step, teams are given the opportunity to restore credit on both the team and individual tests (for the members of their team). As a result, they are highly motivated to engage in a focused restudy of troublesome concepts from the readings.
5. Oral Instructor Feedback. Steps 1–4 enable the instructor to learn of any specific misunderstandings in relation to the key concepts covered in the test. In step 5, he or she provides corrective feedback and instruction aimed at resolving any misunderstandings that remain after the students have done the focused review in preparing their appeals.

Individual Test

The first in-class activity in each instructional unit is an individual RAT (IRAT) on the preclass assignments. The IRATs typically consist of multiple-choice questions that, in combination, enable the instructor to assess whether students have a sound understanding of the *key* concepts from the readings. As a result, the IRAT questions should focus on foundational concepts (and avoid picky details) but be difficult enough to create discussion within the teams (see Appendix A in Michaelsen et al., 2002, 2004 for information on how to create effective IRATs).

Team Test

When students have finished the IRAT, they turn in their answers (which should be scored during the team test) and immediately proceed to the third phase of the RAP, the group RAT (GRAT). During the third phase, students retake the *same test*, but this time the teams must agree on the answers to each test question and immediately check the correctness of their decision using an Immediate Feedback-Assessment Technique (IF-AT) self-scoring answer sheet that provides real-time feedback for the team GRATs. With the IF-AT answer sheets, students scratch off the covering of one of four (or five) boxes in search of a mark that indicates they have found the correct answer. If they find the mark on the first try, they receive full credit. If not, they continue scratching until they do find the mark, but their score is reduced with each unsuccessful scratch. This allows teams to receive partial credit for proximate knowledge (see Figure 2.2).

FIGURE 2.2
IF-AT Answer Sheet

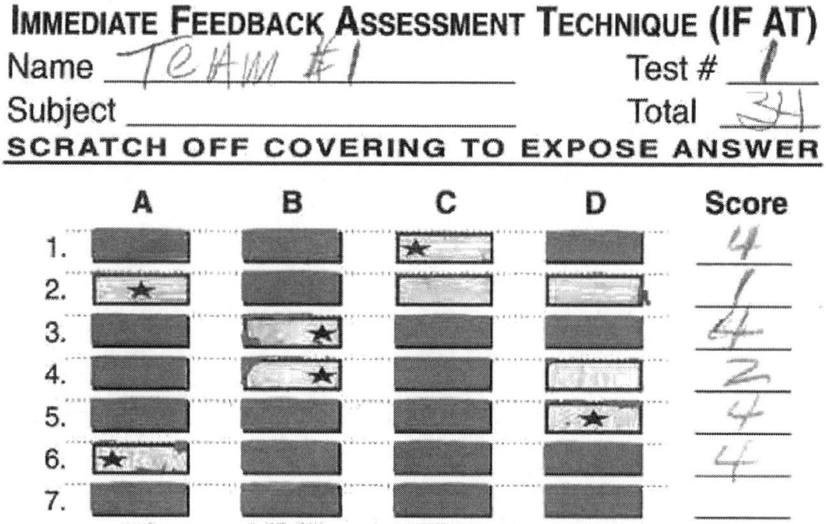

IMMEDIATE FEEDBACK ASSESSMENT TECHNIQUE (IF AT)

Name TEAM #1 Test # 1

Subject Total 34

SCRATCH OFF COVERING TO EXPOSE ANSWER

	A	B	C	D	Score
1.			★		4
2.	★				1
3.		★			4
4.		★			2
5.				★	4
6.	★				4
7.					

In our judgment, the IF-AT answer sheets are the single best way to provide timely feedback on the *group* RATs (not the IRATs, otherwise, members would know the answers before the team test and discussion would be pointless).

Getting truly immediate feedback from the IF-AT provides two key benefits to the teams.

- Truly immediate feedback enables members to quickly correct their misconceptions of the subject matter. Finding a star immediately confirms the validity of their choice, but finding a blank box lets them know they have more work to do.
- Truly immediate feedback creates a situation in which, with no input from the instructor, teams quickly learn how to work together effectively. In fact, IF-ATs virtually eliminate any possibility that one or two members might dominate team discussions. Pushy members are only one scratch away from having to "eat crow," and quiet members are one scratch away from being validated as a valuable source of information and two scratches away from being told that they need to speak up.

The positive impact of the IF-AT on team development is nothing short of astounding. In our judgment, using the IF-ATs with the GRATs is the single most powerful tool one can use to promote learning and cohesiveness in classroom learning teams. Anyone who is not using them already is missing a sure-fire way to increase their effectiveness at implementing TBL.

The IF-AT forms can be ordered from the Web site http://www.epsteineducation .com. When you order a set of forms, they come with different patterns of correct answers; this prevents students from simply memorizing the patterns. The teacher receives a key to find the correct answers on any given set of forms. Further, because they are only used for the *team* tests and can often be used for more than one GRAT, an initial order often covers the needs of several users and/or several years of use. Thus, the cost of the forms is quite reasonable.

Appeals

At this point in the RAP, students proceed to the fourth phase. This phase gives students the opportunity to refer to their assigned reading material and appeal any questions that were missed on the group test. That is, students are allowed to do a focused restudy of the assigned readings to challenge the teacher about their responses on specific items on the group test or about confusion created by either the quality of the questions or inadequacies of the preclass readings. Discussion among group members is usually very animated while the students work together to build a case to support their appeals. The students must produce compelling evidence to convince the teacher to award credit for the answers they missed on the group test. Teachers listening to students argue the fine details of course material while writing team appeals report being convinced their students learn more from appealing answers they got wrong than from confirming the answers they got right. As an integral part of the RAP, this appeals exercise provides yet another review of the readings.

Instructor Feedback

The fifth and final part of the Readiness Assurance Process involves oral feedback from the instructor. This feedback comes immediately *after* the appeals process and allows the instructor to clear up any confusion students may have about any of the concepts presented in the readings. As a result, input from the instructor is typically limited to a brief, focused review of only the most challenging aspects of the preclass reading assignment.

The RAP in Summary

The RAP allows instructors to virtually eliminate class time often wasted in covering material that students can learn on their own. Time is saved because the instructor's input occurs *after* students have (a) individually studied the material, (b) taken an individual test focused on key concepts from the reading assignment, (c) retaken the same test as a member of a learning team, and (d) completed a focused restudy of the most difficult concepts. A cursory review of team-test results illuminates for the instructor which concepts need additional attention so that he or she can correct students' misunderstandings. In contrast to the concerns many instructors express about losing time to group work and not being able to cover as much content, many teachers report being able to cover *more* with the RAP than they can in a lecture. Leveraging the motivational and instructional power of the Readiness Assurance Test leaves the class ample time for students to tackle the application-oriented assignments to develop students' higher-level learning skills.

Beyond its instructional power, the RAP is the backbone of TBL because of its effect on team development. The RAP is the single most powerful team development tool we have ever seen because it *promotes team development* in four specific areas. First, starting early in the course (usually the first few class hours) the students are exposed to immediate and unambiguous feedback on individual and team performance. As a result, each member is explicitly accountable for his or her preclass preparation. Second, because team members work face to face, the impact of the interaction is immediate and personal. Third, since students have a strong vested interest in doing well as a group, they are motivated to engage in a high level of interaction. Finally, cohesiveness continues to build during the final stage of the process, namely, when the instructor is presenting information. Groups become more cohesive because, unlike lectures, the content of the instructor's comments is determined by the results of the RATs and is specifically aimed at providing value-added feedback to the teams.

Even though the impact of the RAP on student learning is limited primarily to ensuring that they have a solid exposure to the content, it is still an extremely valuable teaching/learning activity because it creates a feedback-rich learning environment. By encouraging preclass preparation and intensive give-and-take interaction, this process also increases students' ability to solve difficult problems. Preclass preparation and lively discussion build the intellectual competence of team members and enhance their ability and willingness to provide high-quality feedback to one another. This, in turn, dramatically reduces the teacher's burden of providing feedback to individual students. As a result, the RAP provides a practical way of ensuring that, even in large classes, students are exposed to a high volume of immediate feedback that, in some ways, can actually be better than having a one-on-one relationship between student and instructor.

Promoting Higher-Level Learning

The final stage in the TBL instructional activity sequence for each unit of instruction is using one or more assignments that provide students with the opportunity to deepen their understanding by using the concepts to solve some sort of a problem. As outlined above (and discussed in detail in chapter 3 of this book), good application-focused group assignments foster give-and-take discussions because they focus on decision making (not writing) and enable students to share their conclusions in a form that enables prompt cross-team comparisons and feedback.

Several examples of potential application-focused assignments that meet these criteria are shown in Table 2.2. In each case, the assignment requires teams to use course concepts to make a complex decision that can be represented in a simple form (see chapter 3). As a result, because each of these assignments could be implemented so that teams could receive prompt and detailed *peer* feedback on the quality of their work, the assignments would also enhance learning and team development. Learning is enhanced because students would be forced to reexamine and possibly modify their assumptions and/or interpretations of the facts, and the teams become more cohesive as they pull together in an attempt to defend their positions.

Encouraging the Development of Positive Team Norms

Learning teams will only be successful to the extent that individual members prepare for and actually attend class. Fortunately, if students have ongoing feedback

TABLE 2.2
Examples of Decision-Based Assignments

From a list of two to five plausible, but differentially defensible, outcomes that are related to concepts from the course, have teams choose the one that would be *most* (or least) affected by (plug in an example from the list below):

- A specific temperature increase (in a course in chemistry or botany).
- A drop in the blood glucose level 30 minutes after the administration of a specific drug (in a course in pharmacology or biochemistry).
- A specific cardiac blood-flow pattern (in a course in cardiology).

emphasizing the fact that preclass preparation and class attendance are critical to their team's success, these norms will pretty much develop on their own. One very simple, yet effective, way to provide such feedback to the students is through the use of team folders. The folders should contain an ongoing record of each member's attendance, along with the individual and team scores on the RATs and other assignments (see Appendix D-B1.1 in Michaelsen et al., 2002, 2004). The act of recording the scores and attendance data in the team folders is particularly helpful because it ensures that every team member knows how every other team member is doing. Further, promoting a public awareness of the team scores fosters norms favoring individual preparation and regular attendance because doing so naturally focuses attention on the fact that there is always a positive relationship between individual preparation and attendance and team performance.

Near the End of the Term

Although TBL provides students with multiple opportunities for learning along the way, instructors can solidify and extend student understanding of course content and group process issues by using specific kinds of activities near the end of the term. These are activities that cause students to reflect on their experience during the past semester. Their reflecting is focused on several different areas. In most cases, these end-of-the-semester activities are aimed at reminding students of what they have learned about (a) course concepts, (b) the value of teams in tackling intellectual challenges, (c) the kinds of interaction that promote effective team work, and (d) themselves.

Reinforcing Content Learning

One of the greatest benefits of using TBL is also a potential danger—particularly in health professions schools. Since so little class time is aimed at providing students with their initial exposure to course concepts, many fail to realize how much they have learned that will aid them in taking the board exams. In part, this results from the fact that, based on the reduced volume of lecture notes alone, many medical students are somewhat uneasy and some may actually feel that they have been cheated. As a result, on an ongoing basis—and especially near the end of the course—instructors should make explicit connections between board and end-of-course exams and the RAT questions and application assignments. In addition, an effective way to reassure students is devoting a class period to a concept review. In its simplest form this involves (a) giving students an extensive list of the concepts from the course—especially those that are likely to appear on the board exam, (b) asking them to individually identify any concepts that they don't recognize, (c) compare their conclusions in the teams, and (d) review any concepts that teams identify as needing additional attention.

Learning About the Value of Teams

Concerns about better students being burdened by less-motivated or less-able peers are commonplace with other group-based instructional approaches. TBL, however, enables instructors to provide students with compelling empirical evidence of the value of teams for tackling difficult intellectual challenges. For example, in taking individual and team RATs, students generally have the feeling that the teams are outperforming their own best member, but they are seldom aware of either the magnitude or the pervasiveness of the effect. Near the end of each term, we create a transparency that shows five *cumulative* scores from the RATs for each team—the low, average, and high member score; the team score; and the difference between the highest member score and the team score (see Appendix D, Exhibit D-A7.3 in Michaelsen et al., 2002, 2004). Most students are literally stunned when they see the pattern of scores for the entire class. In the past 20 years, over 99.95% of the teams have outperformed their own best member by an average of nearly 14%. In fact, in the majority of classes, the lowest team score in the class is higher than the single best individual score in the entire class (e.g., see Michaelsen et al., 1989).

Recognizing Effective Team Interaction

Over time, teams get better and better at ferreting out and using members' intellectual resources in making decisions (e.g., Watson et al., 1991). However, unless instructors use an activity that prompts members to explicitly think about group process issues, they are likely to miss an important teaching opportunity. This is because most students, although pleased about the results, generally fail to recognize the changes in members' behavior that have made the improvements possible.

We have used two different approaches for increasing students' awareness of the relationship between group processes and group effectiveness. The aim of both approaches is to have students reflect on how and why members' interaction patterns have changed as their team became more cohesive. One approach is an individual assignment that requires students to (a) review their previous observations about the group, (b) formulate a list of changes or events that made a difference, (c) share their lists with team members, and (d) create a written analysis that addresses barriers to team effectiveness and keys to overcoming them. The other, and more effective approach, involves the same assignment but having students prepare along the way by keeping an ongoing log of observations about how their team has functioned (see Hernandez, 2002).

Learning About Themselves

One of the most important contributions of TBL is that it creates conditions that can enable students to learn a great deal about the way they interact with others. In large measure, this occurs because of the extensive and intensive interaction within the teams. Over time, two important things happen. One is that members really get to know each other's strengths and weaknesses. This makes them better at teaching each other because they can make increasingly accurate assumptions about what a given teammate finds difficult and how best to explain it to that person. The other is that, in the vast majority of teams, members develop such strong interpersonal relationships that they feel morally obligated to provide honest feedback to each other.

Although students learn a great deal about themselves along the way, the instructor can have a significant positive impact on many students' understanding of themselves by using a well-designed peer evaluation process (see chapter 9 in this book). In its simplest form, this involves formally collecting data from team members on how much and in what way they have contributed to each other's learning and making the information (but not who provided it) available to individual students.

Some prefer collecting and feeding back peer evaluation data two or more times during the term (usually in conjunction with major team assignments). Others favor involving teams in developing peer evaluation criteria partway through the term but only collecting the peer evaluation data at the very end of the term. The biggest advantage of collecting and feeding back peer evaluation data along the way is that it gives students the opportunity to make changes. The disadvantage is that having students formally evaluate each other can measurably disrupt the team development process.

PART THREE—BENEFITS OF TEAM-BASED LEARNING

In part, because of its versatility in dealing with the problems associated with the multiple teaching venues in medical education (see chapter 1), TBL produces a wide variety of benefits for students, for medical education administrators, and for individual faculty members who are engaged in the instruction process.

Benefits for Students

In addition to ensuring that students master the basic course content, TBL enables a number of outcomes that are virtually impossible in a lecture-based course format and rarely achieved with any other small-group based instructional approach. With TBL:

1. Most students progress well beyond simply acquiring factual knowledge and achieve a depth of understanding that can only come through solving a *series* of problems that are too complex for even the best students to complete through their individual effort.
2. Virtually every student develops a deep and abiding appreciation of the value of teams for solving difficult, complex and real-world problems.
3. Many students gain profound insights into their strengths and weaknesses as learners and as team members.

4. Compared to a traditional curriculum, introducing TBL enables the at-risk students (probably because of the increased social support and/or peer tutoring) to successfully complete their course work and stay on track in their progress toward graduation.

Benefits From an Administrative Perspective

Many of the benefits for administrators are related to the social impact that results from the fact that the vast majority of groups develop into effective learning teams. With TBL:

1. Almost without exception, the groups develop into effective *self-managed* learning teams. As a result, the faculty and/or professional staff time used for training facilitators and involvement in team facilitation is minimal.
2. Since TBL can be successfully employed in even large classes, the faculty cost of mandated increases in the use of active learning approaches becomes much more of a practical reality.

Benefits for Faculty

There is tremendous benefit for the faculty who use TBL. Because of the student apathy that is a natural response to the traditional lecture-based instruction, even the most dedicated faculty tend to burn out. By contrast, TBL prompts most students to engage in the learning process with a level of energy and enthusiasm that transforms classrooms into a place of excitement that is rewarding for them and the instructor. With TBL:

1. Instructors seldom have to worry about students not being in class or failing to prepare for the work that he or she has planned.
2. When students are truly prepared for class, interacting with them is much more like working with colleagues than with the "empty vessels" that tend to show up in lecture–based courses.
3. Because instructors spend much more time listening and observing than making formal presentations, they develop many more personally rewarding relationships with their students.
4. When the instructor adopts the, "it's about learning *not* about teaching" view of the education process that is a normal outcome of the backward design aspect of TBL, instructors and students naturally tend to become true partners in the education process.

REFERENCES

Bargh, J. A., & Schul, Y. (1980). On the cognitive benefits of teaching. *Journal of Educational Psychology*, *74*(5), 593–604.

Bruning, R. H., Schraw, G. J, & Ronning, R. R. (1994). *Cognitive psychology and instruction* (2nd ed.). Englewood Cliffs, NJ: Prentice Hall.

Fiechtner, S. B., & Davis, E. A. (1985). Why some groups fail: A survey of students' experiences with learning groups. *The Organizational Behavior Teaching Review 9*(4), 58–71.

Hernandez, S. A. (2002). Team-based learning in a marketing principles course: Cooperative structures that facilitate active learning and higher level thinking. *Journal of Marketing Education 24*(1), 45–75.

Michaelsen, L. K., & Black, R. H. (1994). Building learning teams: The key to harnessing the power of small groups in higher education. In S. Kadel & J. Keehner (Eds.), *Collaborative learning: A sourcebook for higher education* (Vol. 2, pp. 65–81). State College, PA: National Center for Teaching, Learning, and Assessment.

Michaelsen, L. K., Cragin, J. P., & Watson, W. E. (1981). Grading and anxiety: A strategy for coping. *Exchange: The Organizational Behavior Teaching Journal 6*(1), 8–14.

Michaelsen, L. K., Knight, A. B., & Fink, L. D. (2002). *Team-based learning: A transformative use of small groups*. Westport, CT: Praeger.

Michaelsen, L. K., Knight, A. B., & Fink, L. D. (2004). *Team-based learning: A transformative use of small groups in college teaching*. Sterling, VA: Stylus.

Michaelsen, L. K., & Schultheiss, E. E. (1988). Making feedback helpful. *The Organizational Behavior Teaching Review 13*(1), 109–113.

Michaelsen, L. K., Watson, W. E., & Black, R. H. (1989). A realistic test of individual versus group consensus decision making. *Journal of Applied Psychology 74*(5): 834–839.

Nungester, R. J., & Duchastel, P. C. (1982). Testing versus review: Effects on retention. *Journal of Applied Psychology 74*(1), 18–22.

Slavin, R. E, & Karweit, N. L. (1981). Cognitive and affective outcomes of an intensive student team-based learning experience. *Journal of Experimental Education 50*(1), 29–35.

Watson, W. E., Kumar, K., & Michaelsen, L. K. (1993). Cultural diversity's impact on group process and performance: Comparing culturally homogeneous and culturally diverse task groups. *The Academy of Management Journal 36*(3), 590–602.

Watson, W. E., Michaelsen, L. K., & Sharp, W. (1991). Member competence, group interaction and group decision-making: A longitudinal study. *Journal of Applied Psychology 76*, 801–809.

Whitehead, A. (1929). *The aims of education*. Cambridge, UK: Cambridge University Press.

Wiggins, G., & McTighe, J. H. (1998). *Understanding by design*. Columbus, OH: Merrill Prentice Hall.

APPENDIX 2.A

Forming Fair Groups Quickly

By Michael Sweet

The following nine steps constitute a simple yet effective way to form heterogeneous but equally talented groups that students see as being fair and that works for classes as small as 10 and as large as 200 or more. The illustration on page 34 provides a visual depiction of how the process unfolds. The nine steps are:

1. **Decide Your Sorting Criteria**

   Ahead of time, decide what characteristics would make the course easier or more difficult for a student. For example, professional experience or previous course work in the field might make the course easier for a student, but having grown up in a different culture and/or having a different native language might make the course experience more difficult.

2. **Prioritize Your Sorting Criteria**

   List these characteristics in order of importance, mixing the "benefit" and "detriment" characteristics together into one list, with the most important characteristic at the top. You must prioritize because many students will have more than one characteristic on your list (e.g., a professional in the field who grew up speaking a different language). Phrase these characteristics carefully, to avoid embarrassing any one group of students. For example, one anthropology teacher uses "did not grow up in Oregon or any of the immediately surrounding states" instead of "speaks English as a second language."

3. **Prepare Your Students**

   Explain to the students that you are going to assemble them into groups and that the process can be a little chaotic, but is also kind of fun. Tell them you are going to ask them to form one long line—around the classroom if necessary—and ask them to carry their belongings with them through the exercise.

4. **Call the First Characteristic**

   Now comes the sorting. Pick your first characteristic, and ask everyone who self-identifies with that characteristic to stand up and begin the line. If it is a characteristic that can be broken down further (e.g., number of years professional experience, number of previous courses in the discipline, distance from Oregon), then ask them to sort themselves as a continuum (most to least, farthest to nearest, etc.). This can provide some nice ice breaking on the fly.

5. **Call the Other Characteristics**

   Now call out your second characteristic, and ask the students to add themselves to the end of the line begun by the first group. Keep doing this until all students are standing in the line. If necessary, your last characteristics can be major and nonmajor, men and women, or some other catch-all categories to make sure everyone winds up in the line.

6. **Count Your Students**

   Once everyone is standing in line, count the number of students in the line. As we all know, the number of students who actually show up is frequently not the number of students our roster says we should expect. So—if class size permits—go down the line and count for yourself so that you will know how many students you *really* have.

7. **Calculate How Many Groups You Want**

   Your students are about to count off to determine which group they will belong to, but you need to determine how high they should count—that is, how many groups there will be in the class. Let's say you have a class of 33 students, and you want groups of 6 or 7. That will give you 3 groups of 7 and 2 groups of 6.

8. **Have the Groups Count Off by the Total Number of *Groups* You Want**

   This is very important and can be confusing: you want to count by the number of groups you want, *not* the number of students you want per group. So with 33 students and a goal of 6 or 7 per group, the students would count off by 5 (not 6 or 7).

9. **Have Group Members Assemble and Introduce Themselves**

   It is easiest if you designate a specific location in the room for each of the groups. Give them a few minutes to introduce themselves, and then get on with class.

A note about the following illustration:
Life rarely provides us with perfect circumstances. You will notice that in the illustrated group formation process, each group ends up with one more of a certain characteristic than any other group. This is bound to happen, as are different group sizes, as students add and drop the course. The best we can do is aim for groups that are as equitable as possible—perfect equality is not realistic.

Step One

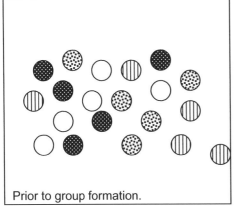

Prior to group formation.

Step Two

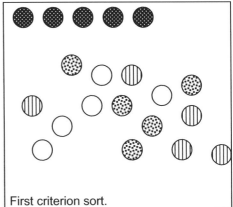

First criterion sort.

Step Three

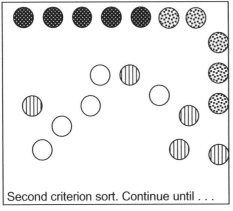

Second criterion sort. Continue until . . .

Step Four

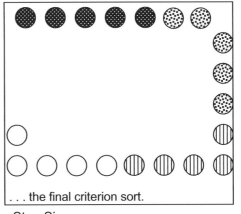

. . . the final criterion sort.

Step Five

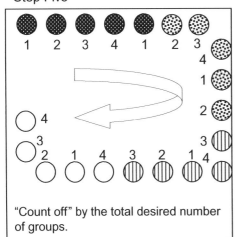

"Count off" by the total desired number of groups.

Step Six

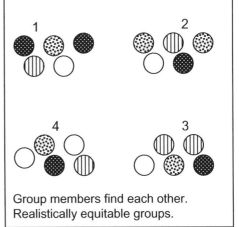

Group members find each other. Realistically equitable groups.

CHAPTER 3

Creating Effective Team Assignments

Larry K. Michaelsen and Michael Sweet

We are often asked, "What is the single most critical aspect of successfully implementing team-based learning (TBL)?" Our unequivocal answer is, "Using team assignments that motivate open, content-related group discussions." If you use good assignments, you will get good results. On the other hand, poor assignment design is the primary cause of most problems encountered by faculty using any form of small-group work (including TBL).

The purpose of this chapter is to delineate the key attributes of effective group/team assignments. Because the nurturing of group cohesiveness is critical to the success of TBL (see chapter 2), we begin by outlining causes and consequences of group cohesiveness in a learning group context. Next, we discuss how different types of assignments (group tasks) affect group cohesiveness and learning. Finally, we present a list of principles that are essential for designing effective group assignments along with a checklist for evaluating the effectiveness of group assignments that can be used in a wide variety of instructional settings and subject areas.

CAUSES AND CONSEQUENCES OF GROUP COHESIVENESS

Cohesiveness is the degree to which members of a group are attracted to each other and are committed to the achievement of group goals. Members of cohesive groups have a strong desire to stay in the group and are willing to make personal sacrifices to ensure the success and/or protect the reputation of the group.

Groups vary in cohesiveness. Furthermore, cohesiveness can change over time, depending on the group's experience. Although cohesiveness is an important dimension in a group's life, a group does not have to be highly cohesive in order to survive. Members of low-cohesiveness groups can live and work together for a long time, but they are not likely to pull together under pressure. While low-cohesiveness groups often survive, highly cohesive groups often *thrive*. Figure 3.1 depicts some causes and effects of cohesiveness.

FIGURE 3.1
Causes and Effects of Cohesiveness

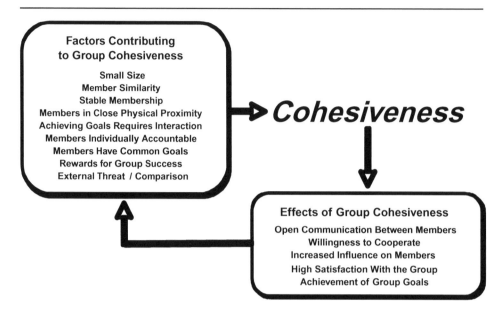

FACTORS CONTRIBUTING TO GROUP COHESIVENESS

A number of factors foster group cohesiveness. Some of the most important are as follows (for an extensive literature review, see chapter 4 in Michaelsen, Knight, & Fink, 2002, 2004):

Small Size

Smaller groups tend to be more cohesive than larger ones. Thus, other things being equal, groups of three or four are more likely to be more cohesive than groups of six or seven. Larger groups tend to have interaction and organization problems. In large groups, subgroups are likely to form and cohesiveness within the subgroups is often higher than for the larger group as a whole. In addition, larger groups often develop formalized procedures as a means of maintaining order. However, formal procedures also tend to limit the extent to which individual members can influence the group. This, in turn reduces cohesiveness and satisfaction with the group.

Group Member Similarity

When people are similar they are more likely to trust each other and share common goals and interests, thus laying a foundation for group cohesiveness. By contrast,

groups with a great deal of diversity (e.g., racial, ethnic, gender, educational background, work, experience, age, etc.) rarely become cohesive unless the potential negative influence of these kinds of differences are offset by other conditions faced by the
group.

Membership Stability

The development of group cohesiveness is a process, not an event. It takes time
and shared experiences for a group to develop a level of cohesiveness that is needed
for the transition from a group of individuals into a team with a sense of collective
efficacy. Further, making any kind of a change in group membership invariably
constitutes a setback to this group development process.

Members in Close Physical Proximity

Being in close physical proximity virtually ensures that group members will at
least begin the team development process by acquiring a set of common experiences.
Further, social eye contact has been shown to trigger the emotional centers of the
brain (Kawashima et al., 1999), giving face-to-face interaction a kind of relationship-
building traction that less direct forms of contact can never achieve.

Achieving Goals Requires Interaction

Group cohesiveness is directly related to group member interaction. Thus, group
assignments contribute to cohesiveness when members *must* interact to accomplish
their work, and group assignments inhibit cohesiveness when the task can be seg-
mented for individuals to work alone on different parts of the overall task.

Members Are Individually Accountable

Cohesiveness is built upon trust among group members. Creating conditions that
encourage individual members to behave in a trustworthy manner starts off the trust-
building process on the right foot.

Members Have Common Goals

Groups only become cohesive when members have one or more common goals.
The more important the common goals are to each member, the higher the
cohesiveness.

Rewards for Group Success

Unless rewards are based primarily on group performance, cohesiveness is likely to be low because individuals are likely to view themselves as simply out for their own gain, or worse, competing with other members of their own group.

External Threat/Comparison

The single most powerful force for the development of group cohesiveness is the presence of an outside force that is perceived to be threatening to members' goals and/or common interests. Differences between members become less important as they pull together to protect themselves, their well-being, and/or their public image.

EFFECTS OF GROUP COHESIVENESS

When the above factors are properly managed, over time the vast majority of groups will develop into real teams and foster the individual member behavior that will enable them to get things done. As groups become more cohesive, the level of trust and understanding among group members increases to the extent that communication patterns change so that even naturally quiet members become willing to engage in intense give-and-take interactions without worrying about being offensive or misunderstood (Michaelsen, Black, & Fink, 1996; Michaelsen, Watson, & Black, 1989; Watson, Kumar, & Michaelsen, 1993; Watson, Michaelsen, & Sharp, 1991). In addition, a primary characteristic of teams (as opposed to groups) is that members see their collective success as integrally tied to their own individual well-being. When this happens, members are highly motivated to invest personal energy into doing group work (Michaelsen, Jones, & Watson, 1993; Shaw, 1981) and members are highly satisfied because the groups become effective in achieving what they have accepted as their own personal goals (see Figure 3.1).

DEVELOPING COHESIVE LEARNING TEAMS

Cohesive learning teams provide an ideal learning environment (see Figure 3.1). Members of cohesive teams willingly complete individual assignments, come to class prepared, and cooperatively contribute to team discussions. However, developing cohesive teams requires careful planning on the part of the instructor. In part, this results from the fact that there are a number of constraints inherent in a classroom environment that explicitly limits a student's ability to make optimal choices with respect to several of the key factors that are required for developing cohesive learning teams (see Figure 3.1).

CLASSROOM SETTING CONSTRAINTS ON TEAM DEVELOPMENT

In most classroom environments, the reality is that the first four factors listed in Figure 3.1 and Table 3.1 present challenges to the development of cohesive learning teams. As a result, we recommend dealing with the situation in the best way possible by keeping membership as stable as possible and groups as permanent as possible (see chapter 2) to offset the fact that some courses (e.g., clerkships) may involve only a few hours of formal classroom work. In addition, we recommend meeting the need for close physical proximity by doing the group work *during* class time and establishing a space for each of the groups (Note: This is especially important in large classes—see chapter 11 in Michaelsen et al., 2002, 2004).

Two other factors, member similarity and small size (see Table 3.1), involve trying to achieve a balance: we want to facilitate team development by using small, homogeneous groups, but we also need to ensure that groups will have the skills and resources they need to succeed by making sure they are large and heterogeneous *enough*. We recommend dealing with these dilemmas by using fairly large (five- to seven-member) heterogeneous groups (see chapter 2).

TABLE 3.1
Classroom Setting Constraints on Team Development

Cohesiveness Factor	Classroom Setting Constraints	Implications for Instructional Practice
Small Size	Larger groups have more/better resources than smaller groups.	Creates a dilemma, limit group resources versus increase difficulty of building teams.
Membership Similarity	Heterogeneous groups have more/better resources than homogeneous groups.	Creates a dilemma, limit group resources versus increase difficulty of building teams.
Stable Membership	Class time for a typical course is about the same as a normal work *week*.	At a minimum, requires the use of permanent groups.
Members in Close Physical Proximity	Only sure face-to-face interaction is *in class*, but in poorly designed rooms.	Musts: (a) use class time for group work, and (b) assign groups to work spaces.
Achieving Goals Requires Interaction	Some tasks require interaction (e.g., deciding) others (e.g., writing) do not.	Must use tasks that maximize discussion and that can't be completed by individuals.
Individual Member Accountability	Developing effective teams requires members to prepare for and attend class.	Requires measuring and rewarding individual preparation and contribution to team.
Members Have Common Goals	Typical common goal is to pass by satisfying course assignments.	Musts: (a) assign group/team tasks, and (b) base part of grade on group work.
Rewards for Group Success	Grades are the primary reward; should be affected by quality of group work.	Must use tasks that enable qualitative (and timely) evaluation of group products.
External Threat/ Comparison	Some tasks facilitate comparison (e.g., deciding) others (e.g., writing) do not.	Must use tasks that enable comparisons of the products created by group work.

We also believe, however, that it is imperative for instructors to do all they can to offset the negative impact that occurs from the fact that medical teaching contexts often require (a) using groups with limited membership stability, (b) teaching in inflexible time blocks and/or in classrooms that make it difficult for groups to work in close physical proximity, and (c) the need for intellectual resources that exist only in fairly large and heterogeneous student groups. Fortunately, in most cases, instructors can still forge a positive outcome by crafting assignments that leverage the remaining cohesiveness factors so that they promote both team development and learning.

OPPORTUNITIES TO PROMOTE TEAM DEVELOPMENT

Three of the six remaining cohesiveness factors (see Figure 3.1 and Table 3.1) involve the course grading system. Instructors can, at least to some degree, ensure that group members have common goals by setting up a grading system in which individual preparation for group work and group assignments both count as part of members' course grades (see chapter 2). In addition, students' motivation to work on behalf of the group is at least partially dependent on the extent to which the rewards (grades) hinge on the quality of the group work.

Without question, however, the greatest opportunity for promoting team development lies in the design of group assignments.

ASSIGNMENTS THAT PROMOTE GROUP COHESIVENESS

Six attributes determine whether a particular assignment will effectively build group cohesiveness:

1. Does it bring members into close *physical proximity*?
2. Does it represent a basis for a *common goal* among team members?
3. Does it promote *individual accountability* among members?
4. Does it motivate a great deal of *discussion* among team members?
5. Does it ensure that members receive immediate, unambiguous, and meaningful *feedback* (preferably involving direct comparisons with the performance outputs from other teams)?
6. Does it provide explicit *rewards* for team performance?

Attribute #1—Promoting Close Physical Proximity

The degree to which a group becomes cohesive is directly related to the extent to which members do things together. Unless *members interact*, groups simply will not become cohesive. Being in close physical proximity virtually ensures that group members will at least begin the team development process by acquiring a set of common experiences. As a result, we strongly recommend using *in-class* group work and avoiding assignments that allow students to complete the assigned task outside class, working individually.

Our experience strongly suggests that requiring groups to do their work outside class creates an overwhelmingly powerful barrier to the development of group cohesiveness. In most cases, the cost of meeting outside class is so great that students will meet only long enough to divide up the work so that they can independently complete the components of the assignment. As a result, they produce a group product in name only and whatever cohesiveness was developed during the initial meeting is usually offset by the worry about whether other members will actually do their part.

Attribute #2—Ensuring That Members Have a Common Goal

This is the easiest to accomplish and the most overrated of the six cohesiveness-building keys. Simply requiring groups to complete an assignment that counts as part of the course grade is a necessary but clearly insufficient step in the right direction. Unless the other factors are also well managed, grading group work can have a powerful negative impact on group cohesiveness (see below). For example, the fact that some students are highly motivated to get an A and others will be satisfied with a C can, in and of itself, have a powerful negative effect on group cohesiveness.

Attribute #3—Promoting Individual Member Accountability

Probably the greatest difference between groups and teams is that teams are able to accomplish more than the sum of individual members' contributions because they are able to (a) motivate *every* member to give his or her very best effort and (b) combine their individual contributions in unique and creative ways. Ironically, one of the most common barriers to team development is when the group does well on an early assignment based primarily on input from one or two confident and able members. When this happens, it often creates a norm that limits contributions from the other group members.

The key to solving this problem is avoiding it in the first place—an ounce of prevention is worth a pound of cure—by using the Readiness Assurance Process (RAP) with Immediate Feedback-Assessment Technique (IF-AT) answer sheets (see chapter 2).

Attribute #4—Promoting Discussion Among Team Members

A great deal of discussion within a group greatly enhances group cohesiveness. Although a number of different types of tasks can produce such interaction, a highly reliable rule of thumb is that assignments increase group cohesiveness when they require members to *make a concrete decision based on the analysis of a complex issue.* A simple way to remember this rule is to visualize the task of a courtroom jury: given a great deal of complex information, the group must work together toward a simple decision—*guilty* or *not guilty*. In the classroom, a common example of this kind of assignment asks students to apply a rule or solve a truly challenging problem. These types of tasks typically require students to use a broad range of intellectual skills that include recognizing and defining concepts, making discriminations, and applying principles or procedural rules (Gagné, 1970). Further, all group members typically have both opportunity and incentive to actively participate in the task because of the genuine need for broad-based member input. The net result is that problem-based tasks almost universally immerse students in information-rich, give-and-take discussions through which their content learning increases. Further, if the assignment is thoughtfully crafted, students are also likely to reinforce two important lessons about group interaction: (a) other members' input is a valuable resource, and (b) *we* can accomplish something by working together that none of us could have accomplished on our own.

Attribute #5—Providing Teams With Meaningful Feedback

A very powerful force for the development of group cohesiveness is immediate, unambiguous, and meaningful feedback. Feedback is particularly powerful when it involves comparing a team's work with the work of other teams that are faced with solving the same problem. The knowledge that any other team has the potential to outperform your team is extremely motivating to students. In fact, the presence of an outside influence that is perceived to threaten individual member goals and/or the well-being of the group, has a significant impact on the outcome of the group (Shaw, 1981). In this situation, the potentially threatening outside influence manifests as the chance of being shown up by other teams in the class. In the scheme of things, this type of influence is quite valuable because differences among individual group members become less important as they pull together to protect themselves and/or their public image from challenges by other teams. As a result, providing performance data that allow comparisons *between* groups is a very powerful tool for increasing group cohesiveness.

Some assignments are clearly better than others at providing such comparisons. In general, the more that assignments provide unambiguous performance feedback, the better they are at promoting team development. Further, the more immediate the feedback, the greater its value to individual learning and group cohesiveness.

By contrast, assignments are likely to *limit* the development of group cohesiveness (and encourage social loafing, or slacking) if they force groups to do the majority of their work in the absence of feedback. When groups have no way of knowing how they are doing (e.g., when groups are asked to produce some sort of a complex product such as a group paper), members are likely to experience a great deal of stress when trying to work with one another. In addition, differences in members' work styles can also produce a great deal of tension in the group. For example, members who have a strong preference for a systematic and orderly approach, grow increasingly anxious as deadlines approach and they often find themselves in conflict with peers who put off their work until the last minute because they feel they work best under pressure.

Attribute #6—Rewarding Group Success

It would be wonderful if students completed group assignments simply for the love of learning. However, most students feel so many pressures on their time that they are prone to be distracted from working on even the most interesting of assignments. Thus, if we fail to create conditions in which doing good group work pays off in some meaningful way, we are, in effect, asking our students to behave irrationally. As a result, teachers have to take on the responsibility for creating a situation in which it actually makes sense for students to work hard to complete an assignment.

The most obvious way to create incentives for members to devote time and energy to group work is to include *group performance* in our grading system. If group work counts, then cohesiveness increases because group members have a clear and concrete reason to work *together*. On the other hand, if students are graded only on their individual work, group cohesiveness will be inhibited by the fact that individuals will correctly see themselves as competing with the other members of their own group.

Rewarding group performance also helps meet the basic human need for social validation. Typically, *everyone* wants to feel he or she can offer something of value to others. Thus, by creating a situation where the output from the group will be assessed, rewarded, and challenged by peers from other groups, we are creating an environment that promotes group cohesiveness and learning.

ASSIGNMENTS THAT REDUCE GROUP COHESIVENESS

What is the *worst* kind of assignment for building group cohesiveness? It would be one with attributes that are the *opposite* of at least the first five of those listed above. Specifically the *worst* kind of an assignment for groups would be one that, even though it was assigned to a group, would cause members to

1. do the group work by working individually.
2. adopt a personal goal of completing only a part of the overall group task.
3. set their own personal performance standards and work pace.
4. limit the amount of discussion with other group members.
5. receive little and/or delayed feedback on the quality of their work—mostly from the instructor (as opposed to other groups).

Few would question that a group assignment with the above attributes would limit learning and the development of group cohesiveness. On the other hand, it is common practice for instructors to use just such an assignment—requiring students to write group term papers. Writing is inherently an *individual activity*—only one set of hands can fit on a keyboard—therefore, the rational way to accomplish the overall task is to divide up the work so that each member independently completes part of the assignment (usually the part that he or she already knows the most about). As a result, after the initial division of labor, seldom, if any, significant discussion and feedback are typically provided until the project has been handed in and graded by the instructor. At that time, it is too late to create either individual accountability or meaningful comparisons with other groups.

Further, when all five of the above attributes are negative, having part of the student's *grade* based on group work is much more likely to be a negative experience than a positive one. Members are well aware that the failure of any member of the group to do well on his or her share of the writing can force the rest of the group members to accept a low grade or engage in a last-minute attempt to salvage a disaster. In fact, high-achieving students often express the feeling that getting an acceptable grade on a group term paper feels like having crossed a freeway during rush hour without being run over. That is an experience that none of us would want to impose on our students but, unless we are careful about the design of our group assignments, that is exactly what we are likely to do.

INCREASING HIGHER-LEVEL LEARNING WITH EFFECTIVE ASSIGNMENTS

The characteristics of group assignments profoundly affect learning and retention because of two different factors. One is that group assignments affect members' exposure to new information because of their impact on group interaction (see above). The other (discussed below) has to do with the fact that the increased openness of peer interactions also has a strong and powerful impact on the cognitive processes through which learning occurs.

HOW WE LEARN

On the surface, when we make reference to what we *know,* we appear to be referring to the sum total of the information we have been exposed to. Taking information in, however, is only part of the learning process (Bruning, Schraw, & Ronning, 1994). Information that is taken in and stored in short-term memory decays very rapidly, and to be useful over time must be transferred to long-term memory. Thus, from a practical standpoint, what we know is only partly a function of the sum total of the information that we have taken in. Information is only useful if (a) it ends up being transferred to long-term memory and (b) we are able to retrieve the information when it is needed.

Impact of What We Know

Our ability to learn is profoundly affected by information we have previously been exposed to and the way this information is stored in our long-term memory. Most importantly, our capability to learn depends on the extent to which the related components of our memory are clustered into well-organized information structures (i.e., sometimes referred to as *schemata*; see Anderson, 1993; Bruning et al., 1994; Mandler, 1984). These information structures are important because they provide hooks that help establish links between new information that is related to what we already know and between the individual components of our existing structures. In addition, these structures provide a backdrop that helps us recognize what we *do not* know (i.e., information that does not fit).

Information Structures and Learning

What we know, then, is largely a function of the number, complexity, and interconnectedness of the information structures in our long-term memory and the information that we are able to retrieve and use. In other words, significant learning has taken place when we increase the amount of information we are able to retrieve and use. This ability to retrieve information usually occurs when new information motivates us to (a) add information to existing information structures, (b) establish new structures, or (c) establish new links within or between existing structures.

Deep Processing

If a learning activity exposes us to new information that neatly connects to one of our existing information structures, then that information is simply linked to the appropriate node in that structure. Educational researcher Jean Piaget (1970) described this process as the simple "assimilation" of new information. However, if new information appears to conflict with existing knowledge, the learning process takes a very different, but even more beneficial, course. Initially, we will search through our long-term memory to review the linkages the apparent conflict is based on. If this review confirms the existence of a conflict, we will be in a state of discomfort until we find a harmonious accommodation. If none is found and the information's credibility is sustained, we are motivated to eliminate the conflict and "accommodate" the new information by modifying and/or adding to existing mental structures. This memory retrieval and examination process is "deep processing" (Svinicki, 2004) and facilitates learning because each stage has a positive impact on our long-term memory. Consequently, an ideal assignment is one that (a) exposes individual learners to credible new information and (b) requires them to reconcile any inconsistencies in their understanding of the new information or between the new information and their own prior knowledge.

Increasing Higher-Level Learning

The importance of exposing students to new information and requiring them to organize and explain it is dramatically illustrated by a series of studies involving learning groups (summarized by Slavin, 1995). In all of the studies, students were divided into four-member "Jigsaw" groups. Each member was assigned to become a subject-matter expert with respect to one of four content areas, and then required to teach that material to the other members of his or her Jigsaw team. In most instances, students in Jigsaw groups scored higher on an overall summative test than students from a control group who had been taught with a more traditional method. The positive benefits of the Jigsaw activity, however, were primarily because of students' mastery of the material they had taught to their peers. Hearing someone else explain a set of concepts (i.e., *listening* to a lecture, which only exposes students to new information) had a minimal positive effect on learning. However, the impact was much greater for the part of the information students had to explain to their peers—a process that forced them to reconcile inconsistencies in their own understanding to answer their classmates' questions.

Two other studies (Lazarowitz, 1991, Lazarowitz & Karsenty, 1990) that involved adding an additional learning task for the Jigsaw groups further illustrate the value of going beyond exposure. After a Jigsaw peer instruction, each Jigsaw team was given a discovery-oriented problem requiring students to actively *use* the information learned and presented by each of four subject-matter experts in the group. The most significant finding from these studies was that requiring students to use the information originally presented by the *other* subject-matter experts on their team increased their long-term ability to recall this information.

Based on the overall results of the Jigsaw studies, it appears that just listening to another peer in a learning group, even when combined with the opportunity to ask clarifying questions, produces only modest gains in long-term memory. On the other hand, assignments that require higher-level thinking skills, such as those involved in teaching others or using concepts to solve problems, produce substantial long-term gains in students' ability to recall and use course concepts.

Other types of learning activities that focus on using higher-level thinking skills have also been shown to produce similar gains when compared to simple cognitive tasks such as listening to lectures or going over one's notes. These include taking tests (Nungester & Duchastel, 1982), writing "minute papers" (Wilson, 1982), and being exposed to opposing views on a subject and then having to resolve the conflict in the process of making a decision (Smith, Johnson, & Johnson, 1981).

In combination, the findings from these studies convincingly argue that the long-term educational impact of group work will be much greater if group assignments go beyond simply exposing learners to new information to requiring *active engagement* in higher-level cognitive skills. As a result, a key to designing assignments that promote both greater depth of understanding and retention is making sure that those assignments require higher-level thinking and problem solving.

CHARACTERISTICS OF EFFECTIVE TEAM ASSIGNMENTS

The preceding sections of this chapter have illustrated the need for assignments that promote high levels of individual accountability and group discussion (both within and between groups). When students are accountable for preparing for group work, they are motivated to *arrive at* the discussions with existing schemata representing their individual understanding of the course concepts and how they relate. When students are thus prepared for group work, the ensuing discussion—both within and between teams—increases learning and retention by exposing them to new information that is often inconsistent with their initial schemata.

THE FOUR *S*s

How does one create assignments that create accountability and foster discussion? We have identified four practical assignment characteristics—fondly referred to as the "four *S*s"—that, in combination, constitute guidelines for creating and implementing effective group assignments. These are (a) assignments should always be designed around a problem that is *significant to students*, (b) all of the students in the class should be working on the *same* problem, (c) students should be required to make a *specific* choice, and (d) groups should *simultaneously* report their choices (Figure 3.2). Further, these procedures apply to all three stages of effective group assignments—individual work prior to group discussions, discussions within groups, and whole-class discussion between groups. The four *S*s are explained in the following paragraphs.

Key #1—*Significant* (to Students) Problem

Effective assignments must capture students' interest. Unless assignments are built around what students see as an interesting and/or relevant problem, most students will view what they are being asked to do as "busy work" and will put forth the minimum effort required to get a satisfactory grade.

Fortunately, unlike many disciplines in which one of the greatest challenges is convincing students that the subject is of value (e.g., history, literature, etc.), instructors in the health professions can establish at least some degree of relevance of their subject matter by building student assignments in a patient diagnosis and/or treatment context. We strongly recommend, however, taking advantage of every opportunity to *emphasize* the patient-care context in the assignment materials. For example, a biochemistry assignment designed around a patient diagnosis or treatment problem will be more likely to be perceived as significant if the data related to the case is presented on lab report forms from a hospital or treatment center where students are likely to work at some point in the near future.

FIGURE 3.2
Four Keys for Creating and Managing Group Assignments

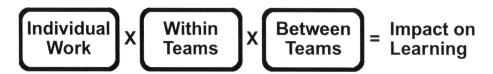

To obtain the maximum impact on learning, assignments at each stage should be characterized by "4s":

○ **Significant Problem**. Individuals/groups should work on a problem that is significant to students.

○ **Same Problem**. Individuals/groups should work on the same problem, case or question.

○ **Specific Choice**. Individuals/groups should be required to use course concepts to make a specific choice.

○ **Simultaneous Report**. Whenever possible individuals and groups should report their choices simultaneously.

Key #2—*Same* Problem

One of the essential characteristics of an effective group assignment is the necessity for discussion *within* and *between* groups. It is through such discussions that students receive immediate feedback regarding the quality of their own thinking as individuals and teams.

In order to facilitate such an exchange, groups must have a common frame of reference. That commonality is derived from working on the same problem, that is, the same assignment/learning activity. Unless everyone is working on the same problem there is no basis for comparison, first between group members and then between groups. Further, having everyone work on the same problem is necessary for students to be able to give and receive peer feedback on their own thinking and their performance as a learning team.

Key #3—*Specific* Choice

As previously discussed, cognitive research shows that learning is greatly enhanced when students are required to engage in higher-level thinking. In order to challenge students to process information at higher levels of cognitive complexity, we must provide them with assignments that create those challenges. We must, as the saying goes, "lead them into situations which they can only escape by thinking."

In general, the best activity to accomplish this goal is to word the assignment in such a way that students are required to make a specific choice. While the terminology may sound vague at this point, in the paragraphs below we provide both several examples of make-a-specific-choice assignments and a rationale on why they work so well in promoting student learning and team development.

Key #4—*Simultaneous* Reports

Once groups have made their choices, they can share the result of their thinking with the rest of the class in one of two ways: sequentially or simultaneously. One significant disadvantage of sequential reporting is that the initial response often has a powerful impact on the subsequent discussion because later-reporting teams change their answer in response to what seems to be an emerging majority view—even if that majority is wrong.

This phenomenon, which we call "answer drift" (Sweet, Michaelsen, & Wright, in press), limits learning and team development for a variety of reasons. One is that it is most likely to occur when the problems being discussed have the greatest potential for producing a meaningful discussion. That is because the more difficult and/or ambiguous the problem, the greater the likelihood that (a) the initial response would be incomplete or even incorrect and (b) subsequent groups would be unsure about the correctness of their answer. Another reason is that answer drift discourages give-and-take discussions because later responders deliberately downplay differences between their initial answer and the one that is being discussed. Finally, sequential reporting limits accountability because the only group that is truly accountable is the one that is forced to open the discussion.

On the other hand, requiring groups to simultaneously reveal their answers virtually eliminates the main problems that result from sequential reporting. For example, in a pharmacology course, a typical assignment would involve requiring teams to choose (from a list of four or five plausible alternatives—see Key #3) what they think would be the best blood-pressure-reducing drug for a patient with a variety of complicating medical problems (including high blood pressure). Then, one simultaneous report option (others will be discussed below) would be for the instructor to signal the teams to simultaneously hold up a card with a number corresponding to their choice. This simultaneous public commitment to a specific choice increases learning and team development because each team is (a) accountable for its choice and (b) motivated to defend its position. Also, the more difficult the problem, the greater the potential for disagreements that are likely to prompt give-and-take discussion.

IMPACT OF MAKE-A-SPECIFIC-CHOICE ASSIGNMENTS

The degree to which assignments stimulate higher-level cognitive skills is largely a function of what we ask students to produce. For example, suppose an instructor of a course in evidence-based medicine wanted to ensure that students were able to understand the diagnostic implications of a wide variety of sources of patient information contained in a patient history file. Three alternative versions of a potential application assignment for an evidence-based medicine course are shown in Table 3.2 (see also Michaelsen et al., 1996, 2002, 2004).

In these examples, the order of the tasks reflects the degree to which each task would require the use of higher-level cognitive skills. For example, alternative number 1 simply asks students to make a list. It is unlikely that this kind of assignment would stimulate higher-level thinking because students could make a list by simply going to a reference source that cites examples of disease process indicators, copying the list and turning it in. With this obvious bit of information in hand, one would readily concede that assignment number 1 is not particularly challenging. Assignment number 2, having to make a choice, is a considerably better assignment. This assignment requires students to critically examine the data in the patient case and decide which diagnosis is most consistent with the pattern of indicators in the case.

While assignment number 2 does require more thinking, assignment number 3, make a specific choice, provides the students with even more practice in using higher-level cognitive skills. Assignment number 3 is better, in part, because students will not be able to complete task number 3 unless they can also complete tasks number 1 and number 2. As is typical with make-a-specific-choice assignments, picking a single indicator that is most critical to making a correct diagnosis will require students to develop and use a number of higher-level cognitive skills. At a minimum, these higher-level skills include making multiple comparisons and discriminations, analyzing content information, and verifying rule application (see Gagné, 1970).

While make-a-specific-choice assignments are beneficial for individual students working alone, these assignments also produce great gains in learning groups. In part, learning increases because make-a-specific-choice assignments provide an additional reason for students to take their work seriously. For example, group interaction provides two additional opportunities to stimulate active learning: the discussion *within*

TABLE 3.2
Wording Assignments to Promote Higher-Level Learning

Make a List

1. List the possible diagnoses that are consistent with the patient data in this case.

Make a Choice

2. Which diagnosis (from a list of five plausible alternatives) is most likely based on the patient data in this case?

Make a Specific Choice

3. Which indicator (from a list of five plausible alternatives) is most critical to making a correct diagnosis in this case?

groups and the discussion *between* groups. When used in a group context, make-a-specific-choice assignments increase learning in each step of the process (a) as students prepare *individually*, (b) as they interact *within* their group, and (c) as they become engaged in the discussion *between* groups (see Figure 3.3). The relative impact of this kind of assignment on each of these situations is discussed in the following paragraphs.

Impact on Individual Preparation for Group Work

Using a series of assignments that require students to make a specific choice enhances individual preparation for group work in three quite different ways. One is that learners have to use higher-level thinking skills in order to actually make a choice. As a result, most will enter the group discussion having made a serious attempt to think through the issues. Second, unless the group is in complete agreement (in which case the assignment is far too easy), members gain additional insight as they prepare to explain the reasons behind their selections to their peers. Third, students' motivation to prepare for subsequent group work is typically enhanced

FIGURE 3.3
Impact of Make-a-Specific-Choice Assignments

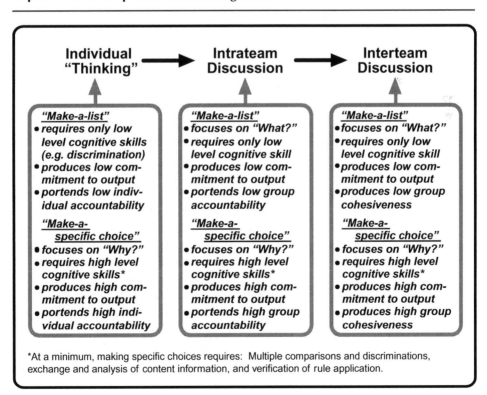

Individual "Thinking"	Intrateam Discussion	Interteam Discussion
"Make-a-list" • requires only low level cognitive skills (e.g. discrimination) • produces low commitment to output • portends low individual accountability	**"Make-a-list"** • focuses on "What?" • requires only low level cognitive skill • produces low commitment to output • portends low group accountability	**"Make-a-list"** • focuses on "What?" • requires only low level cognitive skill • produces low commitment to output • produces low group cohesiveness
"Make-a-specific choice" • focuses on "Why?" • requires high level cognitive skills* • produces high commitment to output • portends high individual accountability	**"Make-a-specific choice"** • focuses on "Why?" • requires high level cognitive skills* • produces high commitment to output • portends high group accountability	**"Make-a-specific choice"** • focuses on "Why?" • requires high level cognitive skills* • produces high commitment to output • produces high group cohesiveness

*At a minimum, making specific choices requires: Multiple comparisons and discriminations, exchange and analysis of content information, and verification of rule application.

because they realize that "make-a-specific-choice assignments" practically eliminate the opportunity to hide and to let someone else carry the group.

Impact on Discussions Within Groups

The difference between make-a-list and make-a-specific-choice assignments is even more evident in intrateam discussions. For example, listing choices that are possibilities tends to be a low-energy team task. One reason for the low energy is that a search for what should be on a list focuses on quantity rather than quality. Another reason is that once several items go on the list, it is easy for quieter and/or less self-assured participants to get off the hook by saying that their ideas are already listed. The last reason is that making a list seldom leads to a feeling of pride in the group output because the majority of the items are likely to be in common with other groups.

By contrast, when groups are asked to select a *single* best choice based on specific criteria and are aware that other groups have been given the same assignment, members are likely to engage in an intense give-and-take discussion regarding why any given choice is better than another. No group wants to be the only one to have made a particular choice and not be able to present a clear and cogent rationale for its position. As a result, most groups will engage in make-a-specific-choice tasks with a great deal of energy. They are also likely to be able and very willing to defend their choices.

Impact on Discussions Between Groups

Group assignments phrased in make-a-specific-choice terms produce their greatest gains in class discussions *between* groups. Two of the benefits arise from the simplicity of the output. We have discovered that assignments that compel groups to make a specific choice invariably promote *group accountability* because any differences between groups are absolutely clear. For example, an assignment that asks groups to select the *most critical indicator* to a correct diagnosis will produce a much more productive between-group discussion than an assignment that asks groups to select a most likely diagnosis (make a choice). Although, in both cases, groups have a vested interest in defending their position to the other groups, comparing most critical indicators (i.e., specific choices) is likely to produce a more intense and informative discussion because the discussion will go beyond simply making a correct diagnosis and focus on the reasons various indicators might be critical to a correct diagnosis.

By contrast, group assignments that produce either lists or nonspecific choices often result in two problems: low-energy class discussion and poor group analyses going unchallenged. The lack of energy results from the fact that groups tend to be far more interested in their own work than that of other groups. Poor analysis often goes unchallenged because (a) having students either make a list or a nonspecific choice is likely to produce so much data that the task of finding something to challenge can be quite difficult, and (b) the absence of clear comparisons allows groups to overlook inconsistencies in their own and other groups' analyses.

Impact of Simultaneous Reporting

Although make-a-specific-choice assignments produce substantial benefits at each of the three stages shown in Figures 3.2 and 3.3, their value is often much greater when the choices are reported simultaneously. This is particularly evident in making the transition from group to total class discussions. Even if students are required to make the same specific decision, having them report sequentially is far less effective than having them report simultaneously. An excellent example of the disparity between the two methods is described below.

After using the RAP, a colleague who teaches physical therapy uses a make-a-specific-choice group assignment to ensure that students can "develop a recovery plan for a patient who has undergone reconstructive knee surgery" (for other examples see Michaelsen et al., 1996, 2002, 2004). He invites a pending or very recently operated-on patient to class, provides his students with the relevant medical records, and gives them the opportunity to ask questions about aspects of the patient's life situation that they think might affect treatment options and/or recovery prognosis. He then asks the teams: "Develop what you think is the ideal treatment recovery plan for the patient you have interviewed." Although the assignment clearly requires students to use course concepts to make a number of specific choices, its impact is greatly enhanced by how he has his groups report their choices.

Effect of Sequential Reporting

For several years, this professor gave Readiness Assurance Tests (RATs), allowed students to use class time to work on the project, and had each of five teams make a 10-minute oral presentation in which students revealed the elements of their treatment plan and the reasons for their choices. After the final presentation, he then opened up the floor for questions and class discussion. With very few exceptions, however, he was disappointed by his students' low energy and shallow analysis of the issues. In part, the problem was that the repetitive nature of the presentations tended to put everyone to sleep, including the instructor. However, the problems did not end there. Differences in the groups' choices—the key to stimulating intergroup discussions—were obscured by several factors. First, the sheer volume of data in five 10-minute presentations made it difficult for students to keep track of all the information. Second, the relevant facts were presented over a 50-minute time span. As a result, the key points tended to get lost in a maze of less relevant commentary. Third, since the groups were likely to use different approaches for representing their analyses, establishing links between key ideas was likely to seem like comparing apples and oranges.

Effect of Simultaneous Reporting With a Poster Gallery Walk

By modifying the assignment by replacing sequential reporting with *simultaneous* reporting, the professor is now much more successful in ensuring that students understand the implications of the choices involved in their treatment plan. Instead of the repetitious sequential reports from each group, he still has them develop their treatment plan in class, but instead of an oral report, he has them create a poster (on a single four-foot-by-three-foot piece of flip-chart paper using 36-point Times New Roman type—so it can be read from a distance—and *without* any way to identify the team that produced it) summarizing each of the key elements of their plan and submit it to him at a specified time before the class period when the plans will be discussed. Then, prior to the start of class, he tapes six *anonymous* treatment plan posters to the classroom wall (five from the teams and one that he has created), and during the class, the teams

1. do a gallery walk (five-minutes or so per poster) to examine the posters and identify
   a. the single best idea from any of the other posters that wasn't on their own poster.
   b. the most glaring Achilles heel on any of the other posters in the form of a question (i.e., one that they don't think the poster owner will be able to answer).
2. record their best idea and Achilles heel question on
   a. a form to be handed in for grading purposes.
   b. a mini poster using a wide felt-tip marker to be used for the simultaneous reports.
3. simultaneously put up their best idea mini poster next to the poster containing the idea, followed by a discussion he facilitates to clarify any questions and/or conflicting choices.
4. simultaneously put up their Achilles heel mini poster next to the poster containing their question, followed by a period of time when the teams formulate answers, then he has the teams report their answer to the question(s), if any, about their poster, and facilitates a give-and-take discussion about the validity of their answers.

The two different reporting options produce dramatically different outcomes. The gallery walk version of the assignment invariably produces a high-energy exchange first within and then between the teams focusing on the strengths and weaknesses of the treatment plans. In contrast to students being overwhelmed with data from 50 minutes of reports, the gallery walk approach ensures that students are exposed to a simultaneous, common, permanent, and highly visual representation of only the essential data: the variables influencing whether a treatment plan (a) is likely to be followed by the patient for which it is designed and (b) if followed, will succeed. Further, the students have a designated time to carefully process and digest the information in an integrated way.

Simultaneous Reporting Alternatives

The key to simultaneous reporting is identifying a simple way to represent the decision (or decisions) involved in solving a complex problem. The simplest and most flexible is having teams hold up a numbered card that corresponds to their choice from a set of alternatives that are under consideration (see Key # 4 above and in chapter 2). Additional gallery walk options we have seen include students creating posters of a concept map (e.g., showing relationships between different types of drugs—and having teams identify the least defensible link on one of the other posters) or flow chart (e.g., showing the pathway through which cells synthesize protein—see McInerney, 2003). Other possibilities for simultaneous reports include summary charts (see chapter 11 in Michaelsen et al., 2002, 2004), overlaying transparencies (e.g., showing the implications of how teams dealt with a series of yes/no decisions or their projected outcomes over time), and using an "answer finder" activity (see the Running Application Exercises video demonstration on http://www.teambasedlearning.org).

In summary, properly designed make-a-specific-choice group assignments with simultaneous reporting virtually ensure a high level of energy in the classroom because of their profound and positive impact on student group cohesiveness. Reaching consensus on a difficult choice requires a great deal of thought and effort. Students, therefore, intuitively realize that differences between teams represent an important source of feedback. Thus, because differences between team choices are so clear, they can represent a significant external threat to a team's self-image, motivating team members to draw together and put forth their best effort.

By contrast, make-a-list assignments seldom promote group cohesiveness because the output is poorly suited for intergroup comparisons. The contrast becomes most apparent when groups share the results of their discussions. Even though groups generally do a pretty good job of making lists, the energy level in the class almost always takes a nosedive when the groups report to the class. In fact, simply getting students to pay attention to each other as representatives go over each item in their respective lists is generally a disheartening experience. Differences that groups might otherwise take pride in and be motivated to defend are both obscured and trivialized by the sheer volume of data.

RECYCLING: A STRATEGY FOR MAXIMIZING THE VALUE OF TEAM ASSIGNMENTS

One of the most difficult challenges faced by medical educators is that there is so much to learn compared with the amount of time students have to learn it. One way to help solve the time problem is by multiplying the value of the application assignments by immediately recycling the same problem, but changing the question so that students will have to look at the facts from a completely different perspective. For example, suppose you had just completed a discussion of the value of various indicators in making a correct diagnosis for a particular patient (see Table 3.2). You could recycle the problem by asking a new question such as, "Which of the following would have the greatest (or least) impact on which factor you would choose as being most critical to making a correct diagnosis?" and then give students a brand new list to choose from (e.g., the patient was perhaps 10 years older, Asian, 30 pounds heavier, female, or diabetic).

Recycling assignments in this way has at least four advantages. First, there is no additional preparation for students and very little additional preparation for the instructor. Second, recycling takes far less class time than starting from scratch with a completely new problem. A third advantage of recycling is that it immediately reinforces the learning that took place in the previous cycle (or cycles). Finally, the richer and more complex the issues, the greater the learning and team-development gains from recycling the problem.

In fact, based on our experience with recycling problems, watching students make and defend their choices enables instructors to discover how to structure the sequence of questions so students can ultimately wind up tackling unbelievably complex problems. The key is gaining an understanding of students' frame of reference so that the instructor can establish a sequence of questions in which each cycle creates a knowledge foundation for the next set of choices. In educational terms, each question creates a scaffold (e.g., see Vygotsky, 1978) that provides a foundation for the next set of choices.

HOW GOOD ARE YOUR ASSIGNMENTS?

Probably the single best indicator of the effectiveness of group assignments is the presence of *task-focused energy* when groups report and compare the results of their work with the work of other groups in the class. When the energy level is high during discussions *between* teams you can be confident that team members have (a) individually prepared in advance for the team work, (b) taken their team work seriously, and (c) increased their ability to tackle even more difficult learning tasks. Good assignments create a high energy level in the classroom and the energy level rises because students are *interested in* and *willing to* spontaneously challenge each other's thinking as well as *defend* their own.

We have observed time and again that the four Ss (*significant* [to students] problem, *same* problem, *specific* choice, and *simultaneous* reporting) have a powerful impact on group cohesiveness and energy in the classroom. Table 3.3 provides a checklist that you can use to preassess the extent to which your assignments incorporate these three procedures.

CONCLUSION

The primary theme of this chapter is to emphasize our belief that good group assignments are absolutely critical for the effective use of TBL as a teaching strategy. In addition, we have offered four specific conclusions about the characteristics of

TABLE 3.3
A Checklist for Effective Group Activities

Prior to Group Discussions:
- Are group members working on the same assignment and required to make a specific choice, individually and in writing?
  (Note: This individual accountability is especially important in newly formed groups.)

During Discussions *Within* Groups:
- Are groups required to share members' individual choices and agree (i.e., reach a group consensus) on a specific choice?
- Will the discussion focus on "Why?" (and/or "How?")
- Will the groups' choice(s) be represented in a form that enables immediate and direct comparisons with other groups*?

During Discussions **Between** Groups:
- Are group decisions reported simultaneously?*
- Do group "reports" focus attention on the absolutely key issues?*
- Are groups given the opportunity to digest and reflect on the entire set of "reports"* before total class discussion begins?
- Will the discussion focus on "Why?" (and/or "How?")

> The more "Yes" answers, the better. If the answer to all eight questions is "Yes," the assignment will effectively promote both learning and group development.

*The form in which individual and group choices are represented largely determines the dynamics of the discussions that follow. Both individual reports to groups and group reports to the class should be as absolutely succinct as possible. *One-word reports are the very best* (e.g. yes/no, best/worst, up/down/no change, etc.) because they invariably stimulate a discussion of why one choice is better than another.

---

good group assignments. First, the vast majority of dysfunctional student behaviors (e.g., free riding, members dominating the discussion, etc.) and complaints (e.g., having to carry the dead wood, the instructor isn't teaching, etc.) are the result of bad assignments, *not* bad students or bad groups. Second, good group assignments can be very effective in promoting students' mastery of basic conceptual material and enhancing higher-level thinking and problem-solving skills. Third, the single best way to gauge the effectiveness of group assignments is to observe the level of energy that is present during the total class discussion stage of the assignment. Finally, assignments that are built upon the foundation of the four Ss will consistently maximize both learning and team development.

REFERENCES

Anderson, J. R. (1993). Problem solving and learning. *American Psychologist, 48*, 35–44.

Bruning, R. H., Schraw, G. J., & Ronning, R. R. (1994). *Cognitive psychology and instruction* (2nd ed.). Englewood Cliffs, NJ: Prentice Hall.

Gagné, R. M. (1970). *The conditions for learning* (2nd ed.). New York: Holt, Rinehart and Winston.

Kawashima, R., Sugiura, M., Kato, Y., Nakamura, A., Hatano, K., Ito, K., et al. (1999). The human amygdala plays an important role in gaze monitoring. *Brain, 122*, 779–783.

Latane, B., Williams, K., & Harkins, S. (1979). Many hands make light the work: The causes and consequences of social loafing. *Journal of Personality and Social Psychology, 37*, 822–832.

Lazarowitz, R. (1991). Learning biology cooperatively: An Israeli junior high school study. *Cooperative Learning, 11*(3), 19–21.

Lazarowitz, R., & Karsenty, G. (1990). Cooperative learning and student's self-esteem in tenth grade biology classrooms. In S. Sharon (Ed.), *Cooperative learning theory and research* (pp. 143–149). New York: Praeger.

Mandler, J. M. (1984). *Stories, scripts, and scenes: Aspects of schema theory*. Hillsdale, NJ: Lawrence Erlbaum.

McInerney, M. J. (2003). Team-based learning enhances long-term retention and critical thinking in an undergraduate microbial physiology course. *Microbiology Education Journal, 4*(1), 3–12.

Michaelsen, L. K., & Black, R. H. (1994). Building learning teams: The key to harnessing the power of small groups in higher education. In *Collaborative learning: A sourcebook for higher education* (Vol. 2, pp. 65–81). State College, PA: National Center for Teaching, Learning and Assessment.

Michaelsen, L. K., Black, R. H., & Fink, L. D. (1996). What every faculty developer needs to know about learning groups. In L. Richlin (Ed.), *To improve the academy: Resources for faculty, instructional and organizational development*. Stillwater, OK : New Forums Press.

Michaelsen, L. K., Jones, C. F., & Watson, W. E. (1993). Beyond groups and cooperation: Building high performance learning teams. In D. L. Wright, & J. P. Lunde (Eds.), *To improve the academy: Resources for faculty, instructional and organizational development* (pp. 124–145). Stillwater, OK: New Forums Press.

Michaelsen, L. K., Knight, A. B., & Fink, L. D. (2002). *Team-based learning: A transformative use of small groups*. Westport, CT: Praeger.

Michaelsen, L. K., Knight, A. B., Fink, L. D. (2004). *Team-based learning: A transformative use of small groups in college teaching*. Sterling, VA: Stylus.

Michaelsen, L. K., Watson, W. E., & Black, R. H. (1989). A realistic test of individual versus group consensus decision making. *Journal of Applied Psychology, 74*(5), 834–839.

Nungester, R. J., & Duchastel, P. C. (1982). Testing versus review: Effects on retention. *Journal of Applied Psychology, 74*(1), 18–22.

Piaget, J. (1970). Piaget's theory. In P. H. Mussen (Ed.), *Carmichael's manual of child psychology* (Vol., 1, 3rd ed., pp. 703–732). New York: Wiley.

Shaw, M. E. (1981). *Group dynamics: The psychology of small group behavior* (3rd ed.). New York: McGraw-Hill.

Slavin, R. E. (1995). *Cooperative learning* (2nd ed.). Boston, MA: Allyn & Bacon.

Smith, K., Johnson, D. W., & Johnson R. T. (1981). Can conflict be constructive? Controversy versus concurrence seeking in learning groups. *Journal of Educational Psychology, 73*(5), 651–663.

Svinicki, M. D. (2004). *Learning and motivation in the postsecondary classroom*. Boston, MA: Anker.

Sweet, M. S., Michaelsen, L. K., & Wright. (in press). Simultaneous report: A reliable method to stimulate class discussion. *The Decision Sciences Journal of Innovative Education*.

Vygotsky, L. S. (1978). *Mind in society: The development of higher psychological processes.* Boston: Harvard University Press.

Watson, W. E., Kumar, K., & Michaelsen, L. K. (1993). Cultural diversity's impact on group process and performance: Comparing culturally homogeneous and culturally diverse task groups. *The Academy of Management Journal, 36*(3), 590–602.

Watson, W. E., Michaelsen, L. K., & Sharp, W. (1991). Member competence, group interaction and group decision-making: A longitudinal study. *Journal of Applied Psychology, 76*, 801–809.

Wilson, Wayne R. (1982). *The use of permanent learning groups in teaching introductory accounting.* Unpublished doctoral dissertation, University of Oklahoma, Norman.

CHAPTER 4

Improving Critical Thinking Skills in the Medical Professional With Team-Based Learning

Herbert F. Janssen, N. P. Skeen, John Bell, and William Bradshaw

Team-based learning (TBL) offers an important alternative to the traditional peda-gogical style used most often in medical education. TBL focuses on learning instead of teaching by placing the student in the spotlight and redefining the role of the professor. The student is required to accept responsibility for preparing before class and is required to participate in group discussions. The opportunity for each student to develop critical thinking skills is embedded in this methodology.

As students prepare for TBL sessions, they must go beyond a simple reading of texts and relying on rote memory. They must ask questions, attempt to apply their understanding, and synthesize the information into a conceptual framework. Such engagement is necessary to empower the student to participate as an active member of the group. The group interaction, then, provides a second opportunity for the student to actively engage the material. Successful completion of the process requires each student to obtain mastery of content and insight into its application.

Developing critical thinking skills in the health professional is a task that has generally been neglected. The need to extend the pedagogy of medical and other health professional schools and programs beyond the traditional lecture has long been recognized but frequently ignored. The Flexner Report (1910) was arguably the most influential early document in shaping the course of medical education in the United States and Canada. It recognized the need to maintain a curriculum that not only stressed scientific content but also taught the use of scientific principles in medical problem solving. It encouraged the use of alternative methods of teaching that required the student to actively construct knowledge and practice its application.

THE FLEXNER REPORT

Abraham Flexner was commissioned by the Carnegie Foundation to investigate and report on the condition of medical education in the United States and Canada.

Supported in part by a U.S. Department of Education Fund for the Improvement of Postsecondary Education (FIPSE), P116B980586, awarded to Brigham Young University.

The report criticized many medical schools for relying too heavily on transferring empirical information and failing to emphasize a scientific approach to education. In particular, Flexner was unimpressed with medical schools that relied on didactic lectures as the primary method of instruction. He strongly supported the use of experimental-based education that encouraged active learning. Flexner stated:

> On the pedagogic side, modern medicine, like all scientific teaching, is characterized by activity. The student no longer merely watches, listens, and memorizes: he *does*. His own activities in the laboratory and in the clinic are the main factors in his instruction and discipline. An education in medicine nowadays involves learning and learning how; the student cannot efficiently know, unless he knows how. (1910, p. 53)

Flexner felt strongly that the teaching model based on transmission of descriptive information had to be modified. He argued that medical education should follow the paradigm of scientific inquiry. In comparing the practice of medicine to scientific investigation he stated,

> The main intellectual tool of the investigator is the working hypothesis, or theory as it is more commonly called. The scientist is confronted by a definite situation; he observes it for the purpose of taking in all the facts, these suggest to him a line of action. He constructs a hypothesis as we say. Upon this he acts, and the practical outcome of his procedure refutes, confirms or modifies his theory. Between theory and fact his mind flies like a shuttle; and theory is helpful and important just to the degree in which it enables him to understand, relate, and control phenomena. This is essentially the technique of research; wherein is it irrelevant to the bedside practice? The physician, too, is confronted by a definite situation. He must (needs) seize its details, and only powers of observation trained in actual experimentation will enable him to do so. The patient's history, condition, symptoms, form his data. Thereupon he, too, frames his working hypothesis, now called a diagnosis. It suggests a line of action. Is he right or wrong? Has he actually amassed all the significant facts? Does his working hypothesis properly put them together? The sick man's progress is nature's comment and criticism. The professional competency of the physician is in proportion to his ability to heed the response which nature thus makes to his ministrations. The progress of science and the scientific or intelligent practice of medicine employ, therefore, exactly the same technique. (p. 55)

He later concludes,

> In methods of instruction there is, once more, nothing to distinguish medical from other sciences. Out-and-out didactic treatment is hopelessly antiquated; it belongs to an age of accepted dogma or supposedly complete information, where the professor "knew" and the students "learned." The lecture indeed continues of limited use. It may be employed in beginning a subject to orient the student, to indicate relations, to forecast a line of study in its practical bearings; from time to time, too, a lecture may profitably sum up, interpret, and relate results experimentally ascertained. (pp. 60–61)

Flexner was not a physician; he was an educator. He worked as a high school teacher and principal for nineteen years before returning to Harvard to continue his studies. His background as a teacher apparently provided him with an appreciation for the elements necessary for any true educational experience. Flexner was critical of schools that operated by disseminating information alone rather than teaching students how to use the information. He fully realized the importance of the scientific method as a tool that was equally useful in the practice of medicine and scientific research. Teaching basic science to medical students was important for content but, more importantly, the methods employed by the scientist provide a working model for the practicing physician.

The scientific method, modified slightly, provides a framework for applying critical thinking in the practice of medicine. This allows the physician, for example, to determine a course of action and reevaluate the patient to determine if the originally selected treatment is working successfully.

Although the Flexner Report was published in 1910, it highlights many of the problems that face medical education today. In general, instruction has continued to overemphasize rote memory and underemphasize active learning during the first two years of basic science education. The amount of medical information available today has provided a wealth of knowledge that far exceeds that of the best-trained medical practitioner of the early 1900s. If Flexner thought that simple lecture should be relegated to the bygone era, what would he think of our system today?

CHANGING THE MEDICAL SCHOOL CURRICULUM

Tests administered by the National Board of Medical Examiners (NBME) have recently shifted away from questions that examine a student's recall of facts to problems that require application of facts to case-based scenarios (Case & Swanson, 2002). These scenarios require background information and understanding of how the data presented in them can be used to diagnose and treat a patient's condition. The case usually includes the age and gender of the patient along with other information, such as lab data, clinical findings, patient history, and so on. Teaching students to solve these problems requires a level of instruction that goes beyond the mere presentation of fact in a traditional lecture format.

Within the last several years the Association of American Medical Colleges (AAMC) has introduced the Curriculum Management and Information Tool (Curr-MIT) program (http://www.aamc.org/meded/curric/start.htm). This program is designed to collect objectives for the curricula at all participating medical schools. When completed, it will allow medical schools to compare curricula, teaching methods, evaluation tools, and so forth. The program stresses the need to develop educational objectives that accurately define curriculum and the manner in which the material will be taught. If we are to keep pace with the changing needs of the students, we must be willing to present the material in a manner that requires critical thinking and provides the students with an opportunity to learn and practice problem solving skills.

The Liaison Committee on Medical Education (LCME) has also stressed changes in medical school curriculum (http://www.lcme.org/functionsnarrative.htm#structure). These changes have accommodated implementation of new teaching styles such as TBL. The LCME has recognized the fallacy of trying to teach problem solving using a curriculum that dates back to a time when professors "knew" and students "learned." In a recent revision of LCME policy it was stated:

> Instruction within the basic sciences should include laboratory or other practical opportunities for the direct application of the scientific method, accurate observation of biomedical phenomena, and critical analysis of data. (2006)

This policy change is consistent with Flexner's suggestion that medical education should include instruction in the scientific method and not be solely content driven. Today, information is readily available through online sources and downloadable textbooks. These advances in technology have decreased the need for providing factual information in the classroom, thus freeing time for approaches, such as TBL, that stress learning and learning how.

WHAT IS IT THAT MEDICAL STUDENTS CAN LEARN HOW TO DO WHILE STILL IN THE CLASSROOM?

In the early 1900s, while Abraham Flexner was criticizing the detached nature of medical education, John Dewey and his wife, Alice, were developing educational methods at the University of Chicago Laboratory Schools. Their philosophy was to teach children by having them engage directly in practical activities that illustrated the principle being taught, namely, learning by doing (Maxcy, 2002). However, Dewey's approach extended beyond merely building intuition by empirically accumulating experience. He saw merit in fostering thinking skills through application of the scientific method, augmenting empirical observation with experimentation and reason (Dewey, 1910).

Dewey practiced his methods by introducing household chores into the classroom of young children (Maxcy, 2002). The equivalent in medical education would be to bring patients, syringes, and scalpels into the medical school classroom for students to experiment with, an act that would be impractical if not forbidden. An alternative that might be viewed as a logical preparation for the time when live contact with patients is permitted is to build experience through the solving of problems at the intellectual level. In the spirit of engaging the problem rather than simply observing it, students should be taught to develop a paradigm of thought that builds deep understanding and becomes the basis for clinical skill later in their training, that is, critical thinking.

Efforts to define critical thinking have pointed to Socrates (Paul & Elder, 2003). His method consisted of a systematic use of well-formulated questions to evaluate beliefs and assess the feasibility of inferences. This philosophy remains the basis for contemporary models of learning and thought. Advocates of critical thinking have expanded the pedagogical styles of earlier writers; however, many of the same approaches remain. These include active participation of the learner in the educational process, following a logical sequence in the decision-making process, basing conclusions on truths instead of beliefs, considering all acceptable options, developing and applying solutions, and continually reapplying the process as new questions arise.

Fogler and LeBlanc (1995) described a problem-solving strategy based on a five-step progression that closely resembles the scientific method. According to their scheme, the steps in creative problem solving are as follows:

1. The problem is initially defined.
2. Several solutions are generated.
3. One solution is selected.
4. The solution is implemented.
5. Success is evaluated.

They emphasize the importance of carefully considering each step before moving to the next. One cannot hope for an outcome that is any stronger than the most flawed step in the process. For example, if the real problem is not correctly defined in the first step, subsequent efforts become irrelevant, and failure is assured. The authors encourage continued evaluation of the entire process to help ensure ultimate success.

Paul and Elder (2003) have defined eight elements involved in the process of thought. They suggest that careful analysis and self-awareness regarding those elements improve the quality of thought used to address any issue. These elements are as follows:

1. A well-defined purpose should be clearly stated so that it will not be confused with a related but different purpose. As the analysis progresses, care should be taken to insure that the process has remained on task and not strayed from the desired target.
2. The question to be addressed must be identified and articulated carefully and, if necessary, be subdivided into questions that can be more easily resolved.
3. All thinking involves assumptions. These must be clearly recognized and justified or eliminated.
4. The solutions generated undoubtedly reflect a particular point-of-view. In an attempt to keep this from becoming a stumbling block, the views of others should be sought and carefully considered. Otherwise, feasible solutions that could have produced viable alternatives will be ignored.
5. Informed decisions are dependent on data and information gathered from a variety of sources. Verifying the accuracy of this information is critical. One should

include all data whether or not it supports or refutes some predetermined point of view. Failure to do so results in intellectual dishonesty.

6. The concepts and theories relevant to the issue under consideration must be identified and clarified.

7. If the analysis is successful, it will generate conclusions. However, some conclusions may be less than optimal. Care should be taken to avoid the conclusion that is accepted only because everyone is tired of thinking.

8. Solutions have implications. The challenge of critical thinking must include a careful evaluation of its ultimate consequences. These may include negative and positive implications, and both must be considered. (p. 2)

Critical thinking requires that careful attention be paid to each element to prevent the pitfalls of egocentric thought and to indicate potential problems. For example, if a thinker fails, either consciously or subconsciously, to consider valid information because it runs contrary to his or her original belief system, the final results of the critical thinking process will be flawed. A review of the thought patterns articulated by these authors provides insight into the process of problem solving and how individuals might be able to improve that process for themselves.

SOME PRACTICAL IDEAS FOR FOSTERING CRITICAL THOUGHT IN THE MEDICAL SCHOOL CLASSROOM

It is reasonable to ask whether the various resources available for training of medical students are being used as effectively as possible. A number of those who teach the basic preparatory science courses will admit to feeling underused when their work consists almost entirely of rehearsing for an hour or two the same factual information that a conscientious student could acquire from a careful reading of a chapter from a textbook. A paradigm shift is suggested here, in which responsibility for obtaining the foundational language, facts, and concepts is delegated to individual students before class, and teachers use classroom time to promote analytical thinking skills through pedagogical techniques that permit the transfer of that information to medical practice. Both students and teachers perform the tasks they are best suited to.

Consider a learning paradigm that consists of four basic components. First, students acquire the basic facts through reading of texts. As in other applications of TBL, their acquisition of the facts is assessed through individual and group Readiness Assurance Tests (RATs). Second, students process and apply their understanding through solving relevant authentic problems as a team. Third, students assess their understanding and receive feedback. Fourth, the process is repeated to develop deep understanding. The TBL approach described elsewhere in this volume provides specific details about how to make this paradigm functional. The issue that may require the most thought and preparation on the part of the instructor is development of appropriate problems. For medical education, the obvious application is the interpretation of scientific and/or clinical data for diagnosis and treatment of pathological states. Depending on the scenario used and the topic addressed, the problems may require greater flexibility in terms of the types of responses expected than is typically allowed in the TBL structure. Here are two examples of the types of items that could be used.

1. It is well recognized that elderly individuals often fail to consume adequate quantities of water. It has also been noted that elderly individuals are constipated. What is a logical explanation connecting these two observations? In your explanation, make reference to hormonal control mechanism that may be important in this scenario.
2. Mrs. Jones is a 57-year-old white female who presents at the Internal Medicine Clinic following referral by her primary care physician. She complains of dry mouth, frequent urination, and low levels of energy. Physical examination reveals:

Height: 64 inches
Weight: 185 pounds
BP: 160/110

Blood and urine were collected for stat labs. Results were:

Analysis	Plasma mg/dL	Urine mg/dL
Na+	140	200
Cl-	105	
K+	4.6	
Glucose	225	200
Creatinine	1.0	150
BUN	10	100
Hematocrit	45%	
Urine volume		1.5ml/min
Protein	1+	

Her referral to you requests your assistance in selecting the best diuretic for this patient. Your task is to suggest the proper medication for this patient and justify your choice.

One approach to using team-based problem-solving strategies in the classroom would be to simply confront the students with the problem and let them proceed by a process of trial and error. This approach has the merit of allowing students to discover useful strategies that are personal and therefore directly applicable to each individual student. However, students will vary widely in their ability to generate productive strategies intuitively. It will be time consuming for all, frustrating for many, and completely ineffective for a few. More insidiously, it may allow some students to develop flawed strategies that are reinforced by temporary successes leading only to tears and malpractice suits down the road. A superior plan is to provide an established framework for systematic, logical thought that students can then explore and adapt to their own abilities.

The following represents one possible framework amenable to the medical school classroom. This scheme is an adaptation of the traditional scientific method using elements of the principles taught by Paul and Elder (2003). It fits the clinical setting because it is designed to accommodate the variations that exist when a situation cannot be controlled to meet the rigors imposed by scientific investigation. It consists of seven steps:

1. Define a purpose.
   One might initially suppose that this step is trivial: cure the patient of the disease. In fact, the physician is often faced with a variety of potential objectives in formulating a treatment plan depending on the needs of individual patients and the nature of their conditions. For example, a patient with inoperable cancer may sign a "do not resuscitate" (DNR) order and wish only to be kept comfortable, while another patient may wish to explore all treatment options. Obviously determining a clear goal will drastically alter the remaining steps that should be followed in the individual's care.

2. Formulate questions.
   This is an important step that can easily be ignored as one rushes to a diagnosis and treatment plan. However, failure to ask the appropriate question(s) can easily lead to inadequate information, misdiagnosis, and flawed treatment. Certain questions should always be asked: "What information is needed to make a correct diagnosis? What alternative explanations might also account for the clinical findings? What tests would allow the various explanations to be excluded? What assumptions am I making? Are they valid?" Other questions will vary based on the goal or purpose previously determined. In the first scenario mentioned above, the physician must answer the question, "What is the best treatment for pain management for the patient?" In caring for the second patient, the physician must ask the question, "What cancer treatments are available for this individual?"

3. Obtain information.
   There are several issues with respect to the information used to make a correct evaluation of a patient's condition. Dealing with these issues is a critical aspect of the classroom experience in the basic sciences. The first concern is the type of information to be accessed. At least three categories ought to be included in the students' repertoire: that in the published literature, that which they have acquired as part of their background, and data from clinical tests. Second, students should be required to wrestle with the enormity of the repertoire, distinguishing what is relevant from what is extraneous. Third, they must evaluate the accuracy of the information. Fourth, they must assess whether the body of

information they have chosen to include is complete or whether additional sources should be consulted.

The information available to the medical community has expanded greatly and the rate of expansion is increasing rapidly. Fortunately, the same technology that has propagated the rapid accumulation of information has also helped provide easier access to literature. Using a handheld computer, the physician can wirelessly access the vast wealth of information stored in textbooks and journal articles. Information that medical students were once required to memorize is now either obsolete or can be gained electronically at the patient's bedside. Teaching students how to use this information to solve problems is a much more productive use of classroom time.

4. Propose an effective solution justified by the information.
This is the element that is usually most challenging for students to learn. Some are able to rely on innate abilities or prior experience while others struggle and feel frustrated when their peers seem to be more successful. Experience dictates that one cannot teach logical reasoning per se and expect students to then transfer a set of rules or an understanding of deductive and inductive logic to solving of medical problems. Simply put, one cannot endow students with an algorithm for drawing logical conclusions from data. Instead, they must practice repeatedly and search for their own algorithm. The process is expedited by having a coach to provide frequent feedback and encouragement. The instructor is clearly the appropriate person to function as this coach. Since professors will be unable to reach every student adequately, they must find a way to clone themselves. This can be accomplished in large part by encouraging students to interact productively and take advantage of each other's expertise. Hence, the TBL approach becomes invaluable. The instructor must be wise, however, to train the students in how to interact and be helpful rather than dominate and ignore.

5. Learn the outcome of the proposed solution.
The instructor must be prepared with a full range of likely outcomes to match the variety of solutions that students will propose. If every student proposes the ideal solution, the instructor should consider generating more complex problems.

Students will develop their thinking skills better if they receive authentic feedback in the form of patient outcomes without editorial comment than if the instructor corrects or amends their solution for them.

6. Adjust the proposed solution based on patient outcomes.
The uniqueness of each patient demands that he or she be viewed as a separate case. In the scientific setting, the researcher reproduces the experiment and is ethically bound to accept and report the results as they appear. The physician is under no such obligation and is duty bound to reexamine the patient and adjust the treatment in an attempt to achieve the desired goal. If reevaluation suggests an adjustment in treatment is needed, the physician must reenter the critical thinking cycle to determine when the intervention should occur and how it should be implemented. It is possible that the goal of treatment has changed as the disease process developed. For example, if the disease has progressed unabated

by the current treatment, the patient may elect to sign a DNR order. If this occurs, a new question will need to be asked and new solutions developed. In this case, therapies designed to cure the disease will be replaced by those designed to provide comfort and relieve pain. Other alterations in patient treatment may be necessitated as new test results become available and/or new diagnoses made.

7. Reflect, evaluate, and plan how the next problem might be handled better.
   The sequence of steps suggested above constitutes a learning cycle that should be repeated frequently. It is very useful at the conclusion of each round of problem solving to review the process, note when the proposed plan of action succeeded, and especially to correct misconceptions or misreading of data or misapplications of treatments.

THE ROLES OF THE INSTRUCTOR AND STUDENTS

As mentioned earlier, TBL is an excellent pedagogical method for implementation of critical thinking strategies. The emphasis placed on student-focused education and group interaction provides an opportunity for directed practice in problem solving (Michaelsen, Knight, & Fink, 2002, 2004). Furthermore, in this learning model the professor's and students' roles have been drastically altered. Instead of using preparation time to carefully script elaborate presentations and fabricate slides, the instructor must spend that time making decisions about what the students will do. The following are some of the obvious tasks to be accomplished before class begins:

- Make responsible content decisions. Few professors are at risk of including too little. The more common practice is to include excessive detail that, while interesting to the professor, often obscures the truly important concepts and leaves inadequate time for students to process and apply the foundational information.
- Decide how students will ultimately be evaluated on that content and the application thereof. Design exam items now to guide one's thinking through the rest of the pedagogical plan. This is the time to ensure that there is a good match between the objectives of the course and the assessment on the final exam. If the goal is to foster critical thinking skills in a clinical setting through TBL practices, traditional multiple-choice items that primarily require recall of factual information will not suffice. The more difficult task of designing exam items that require analytical reasoning will be required.
- Choose appropriate reading assignments. These must be sufficient to prepare students well on the necessary content. However, if the assignment is too lengthy with irrelevant detail, students will become discouraged and/or decide that the reading assignments are not really important.
- Build meaningful RATs that focus less on factual recall and more on conceptual understanding.

- Identify clinical applications (problems) relevant to the content topic.
- Anticipate both high- and low-quality solutions to the application and prepare authentic patient outcomes for each.
- Develop strategies for coaching students through steps of the problem-solving process, promoting equitable group participation, and teaching effective reflection and evaluation techniques.

The students' role is symmetrical with that of the instructor. If the instructor is now a coach and designer rather than presenter, the student must become an active participant rather than observer:

- Acquire foundational information from the text before class rather than depend on the instructor to filter the important information from the peripheral details.
- Become independent in constructing a meaningful conceptual framework. Students generally favor a lecture for gaining the information because the instructor has already completed this task. In this new paradigm, the student must accept this responsibility even though more work will be required. It may be beneficial to remind students that the effort they expend now will pay dividends at the end of the term when they traditionally engage in lengthy yet fruitless cramming sessions.
- Be a willing participant on the team.

During individual preparation, the students should be expected to evaluate the available literature rather than accepting all information at face value. This would be especially true if the readings include information published in the medical literature. Quite frequently, literature can be found that presents different views on the same topic. For example, authors may express different opinions on the effectiveness of a drug in the treatment of a specific disease. Similar differences of opinion often exist in how a certain disease condition should be diagnosed, treated, or handled in long-term follow-up. Having students discuss the validity of a single case report compared to a well-conducted multicenter clinical trial will be useful. Such differences can be emphasized during the individual RAT by asking probing questions that challenge students to not only answer but also defend the validity of their answer as opposed to other possibilities. These same probing questions will also permit students to develop critical thinking skills in the group RAT. During the group interaction, students should be expected to follow the "elements of thought" set forth by Paul and Elder (2003). This will help guide the group away from agreeing with the dominant personality in the group and will encourage the group to consider everyone's opinion based on intellectual merit. It should also encourage students to question their own assumptions, points of view, concepts, and conclusions. Here again, asking students to consider alternative solutions would help them develop a greater appreciation for the opinions of other group members.

RELEVANCE BEYOND THE MEDICAL SCHOOL CLASSROOM

The Accreditation Council for Graduate Medical Education (ACGME) evaluates and accredits medical residency programs in the United States (http://www.acg me.org/acWebsite/home/home.asp). The 28 residency review committees assess each program based on preestablished standards. Over the last several years, the ACGME has established six core competencies that set basic conditions for all residency pro grams. Residency programs are required to demonstrate their ability to train residents in each area. Residents are likewise required to demonstrate that they have compe tency in each area. The six core competencies go beyond the basics of patient care and medical knowledge. Professionalism and communication skills, along with systems-based practice and practice-based learning and improvement have increased the complexity of resident training. The critical thinking skills that should be taught in undergraduate medical school are now required to complete residency training. Competency in systems-based practice requires the physicians to interact with other medical professionals to achieve the best outcome for their patient.

CONCLUSION

Improvement in medical education might profitably begin with a vision of the classroom as an effective venue to foster critical thinking skills instead of merely the setting to present information. Although the formal elements of thought and the process of scientific inquiry have been defined, a didactic review of those elements will never improve the ability of students to apply them. Development of skill in logical reasoning, especially as related to the clinical application of medical science, happens best under the tutelage of frequent directed practice. In this model instruc tors become coaches who, having designed demanding in-class problem-solving exer cises, are adept at monitoring student performance and providing feedback to improve their learning behaviors. Moreover, students cease to function as passive note takers, anticipating a future time when they will need to thoughtfully apply basic scientific concepts in restoring health to their patients. TBL is one effective template through which these reforms might be realized.

REFERENCES

Case, S. M., & Swanson, D. B. (2002). *Constructing written test questions for the basic and clinical sciences* (3rd ed.). Philadelphia: National Board of Medical Examiners.

Dewey J. (1910). *How we think*. Lexington, MA: D. C. Heath.

Flexner A. (1910) *Medical education in the United Stated and Canada*. Bulletin number four. (The Flexner Report). New York: The Carnegie Foundation.

Fogler, H. S., & LeBlanc, S. E. (1995). *Strategies for creative problem solving*. Upper Saddle River, NJ: Prentice Hall.

Liaison Committee on Medical Education. (2006, February). LCME Accreditation Standards. Retrieved from http://www.lcme.org/functionsnarrative.htm#structure

Maxcy, S. J. (Ed.). (2002). *John Dewey and American education*. Bristol, UK: Thoemees Press.

Michaelsen, L. K., Knight, A. B., & Fink, L. D. (2002). *Team-based learning: A transformative use of small groups*. London: Praeger.

Michaelsen, L. K., Knight, A. B., & Fink, L. D. (2004). *Team-based learning: A transformative use of small groups in college teaching*. Sterling, VA: Stylus Publishing.

Paul, R., & Elder, L. (2003). *Critical thinking: Concept and tools. The foundation for critical thinking* (3rd ed.). Dillon Beach, CA: The Foundation for Critical Thinking.

CHAPTER 5

An Educational Rationale for the Use of Team-Based Learning

Didactic Versus Dialectic Teaching

Herbert F. Janssen, N. P. Skeen, R. C. Schutt, and Kathryn K. McMahon

Many new trends in education have been introduced and used during the past four decades. These have included (but are certainly not limited to) (a) the use of educational objectives, (b) core curriculum, (c) enhanced audio visual techniques, (d) programmed textbooks, (e) team teaching, (f) computer-aided instruction, and (g) learning portfolios. All of these have claimed to improve learning; however, many have fallen from their initial acceptance and have been replaced with more recent fads in education. Why do we have this continual turnover in educational approaches? While the answer is not always clear, it appears that lasting techniques focus on the learner instead of the educator, and on the process rather then the content.

Team-based learning (TBL) is a recent addition to the pedagogical approaches used in medical education. What does this technique offer that separates it from other approaches used in the past?

TEACHING IN MEDICAL SCHOOLS

Medical schools of all places should stress the development of a student's learning process. It appears obvious that the symptoms and treatment for each patient will be somewhat different. Rarely will any two patients have a routine textbook case presentation. As a result, medical school education should prepare the students to adapt to each new situation rather than memorize how a disease process appears in the classical "70 kg man" that exists only in the physiology textbook.

The Flexner (1910) report recognized that medical education should teach students to use problem-solving techniques instead of simply to learn content by rote memory. Flexner proposed to accomplish this by promoting active learning and

Supported in part by a U.S. Department of Education Fund for the Improvement of Postsecondary Education (FIPSE) grant, P116B980586, awarded to Brigham Young University.

hands-on practical experience rather than traditional lectures. According to Flexner, didactic teaching in a lecture hall should be reserved for the introduction of new material or the presentation of summary material near the end of a section. Once the physician was in the clinic, he proposed that the physician should address the patient's medical condition using steps similar to those used by the scientist. The lab data and patient's progress would confirm or refute the initial diagnosis and suggest alterations in treatment protocol.

Recently the Liaison Committee on Medical Education (LCME) reaffirmed Flexner's recommendations. The new accreditation standards indicate that medical schools must teach students to "collect or utilize data to test and/or verify hypotheses or to address questions about biomedical principles and/or phenomena" (LCME, 2007). This recent alteration in accreditation standards indicates the recognition that we have to shift from a content-driven curriculum (didactic) to one that teaches thought processes (dialectic). The recognition that the scientific method is an important tool for the medical practitioner is a significant step forward for the medical school accreditation process, even if it is finally being implemented almost a century after it was originally suggested.

Didactic Teaching

Didactic is defined in medical terms as "conveying instruction by lectures and books rather than by practice" (Barnhart, 1872). It is derived from the Greek word *didakikos* meaning "apt at teaching" (Taylor, 1974). As the Greek word implies, the focus is on teaching not learning. During the last century, medical education has moved more to the use of didactic teaching as its primary method of instruction. This method focuses the educational process on the instructor. In this setting, the student can memorize content without having to engage the information at a level needed to truly understand its practical application. A somewhat sarcastic definition of didactic instruction states, "Information is transferred from the notes of the lecturer to the notes of the student without passing through the mind of either." In this transfer little or nothing occurs that improves the students' understanding of the material.

Didactic teaching makes the assumption that the professor is correct and the students cannot question the information. Often little time is allowed for students to question the authority of the instructor. This type of teaching encourages complacency and replaces curiosity with the desire to achieve a higher grade instead of a higher level of knowledge. Students assume that their ability to recall facts is equivalent to a true understanding of the material. Students learn to accept an instructor's point of view and mistakenly assume they have gained independent knowledge without having to mentally engage the material. This type of teaching is similar to cult indoctrination that controls cult members by demanding adherence to the doctrine provided to them by the leader. When coupled with sleep deprivation and fatigue, the individual (student or cult inductee) loses any interest in pursuing additional knowledge or thinking independently. Professors, who attempt to teach logic and reasoning skills, must first undo the student's preconceived notion that rote memory is equivalent to learning and understanding. Reasoning skills can only be taught after the student rejects the notion that memorization is equivalent to true knowledge and embraces the need to actively engage the material from one's own point of view.

Previous researchers have clearly demonstrated that didactic teaching is limited in its usefulness. John Dewey recognized the need to teach students the ability to think. While reviewing the shortcomings of teaching facts without thinking ability he stated, "And skill obtained apart from thinking is not connected with any sense of purpose for which it is to be used. It consequently leaves a man at the mercy of his routine habits and of the authoritative control of others, who know what they are about and are not especially scrupulous as to their means of achievement" (Dewey, 2002).

Humbling information for the professor who steadfastly holds to the use of the lecture can be found in the following research:

1. During lecture, students are not attending to what is being presented 40% of the time (Pollio, 1984, p. 11).
2. Students retain 70% of the material in the first 10 minutes of a lecture and 20% in the last 10 minutes (McKeachie, 1986, p. 72).
3. Students lose their initial interest and attention levels continue to drop as a lecture proceeds (Verner & Dickinson, 1967, pp. 85–90).
4. Four months after taking an introductory psychology course, only 8% have more information than a control group that never had the course (Rickard, Rogers, Ellis, & Beidleman, 1988, pp. 151–152).

Lujan and DiCarlo (2006) argue that there is entirely too much content being taught, thus inhibiting the student's ability to actively think about the material presented in the curriculum. Two main goals of the professional school education are to prepare the student to pass the licensure exams and to function as independent thinkers in their clinical practice. Teaching students using a curriculum based on rote memory accomplishes neither.

Dialectic Teaching

The word dialectic comes from the Greek word *dialektike* meaning "art of reasoning." Dialectic is defined as the art or practice of logical discussion employed in finding out the truth of a theory or opinion (Taylor, 1974).

In about 400 BC, Socrates introduced an approach that continually reappears as one of the most influential educational strategies ever used. He is remembered primarily for *how* he taught rather than *what* he taught. His approach of answering a question with a question required his students to evaluate any response they provided and reevaluate their viewpoint based on opinions and information provided by others. They were required to produce a logical rationale for each statement they made and consider the effect it might have if implemented as they proposed.

The Socratic method of teaching focuses on the student, requiring one to think independently and to examine and reexamine each assertion. Each individual is required to carefully examine the logic of each statement and to reevaluate that logic based on input from other individuals and other sources. The leader provides questions rather than answers. These continually refocus the group toward an ultimate conclusion that can stand the test of logical examination. This approach has become known as Socratic dialogue and is based on the use of questions rather than answers to stimulate discussion. The method is called dialectic, from the Greek, meaning "art of debate." Socrates' development and use of the technique has established him as one of the greatest educators of all times, not for what he taught but for altering the thought patterns of the students. While he helped direct the discussions, the student's ability to engage the topic and logically address each issue was the ultimate goal.

This teaching/learning paradigm helped each person develop a process of thought that could be used throughout a lifetime. Socrates reportedly referred to himself as a midwife, not producing ideas by himself but drawing them from the minds of his students (Mannion, 2002).

Kant (1781/2003) stated,

> Without sensibility no object would be given to us, without understanding no object would be thought. Thoughts without content are empty, intuitions without concepts are blind. It is, therefore, just as necessary to make our concepts sensible, that is, to add the object to them in intuition, as to make our intuitions intelligible, that is, to bring them under concepts. These two powers or capacities cannot exchange their functions. The understanding can intuit nothing, the senses can think nothing. Only through their union can knowledge arise. (p. 93)

Dewey believed that reflective thinking should be a significant outcome of the curriculum and the teaching-learning process (Axtelle & Burnett, 1970).

DIALECTIC TEACHING WITH TBL

Dialectic instruction is an integral part of TBL. TBL also incorporates the other pedagogy approaches that, when combined, offer the student an excellent opportunity to learn the content and also learn a process. Both play an important role independently, but when combined they can help the student develop success in a specific discipline and also develop lifelong learning skills.

Prior to coming to the TBL session, the student is required to review all material provided in handouts, textbooks, and so forth. In the classroom, the student will take the individual Readiness Assurance Test (IRAT) (Michaelsen, Knight, & Fink, 2002), which provides the student with a formative evaluation of the information the student learned independently. It also provides an instructor with an evaluation of how well students were able to gain information on their own. Following completion of the initial test, the students are provided with questions they work on as a group. During the group discussion, the students learn important dialectic skills expressing their own points of view and considering and evaluating the viewpoints of others. The dialectic portion of TBL also allows latitude in the thought process, providing an opportunity for the individual to add new information, new ideas, and so on. As such, the exchange of ideas is not a conclusion but a process in developing each individual's own reasoning skills.

The mental process of the student does not stop when the evaluation of the ideas are complete. Instead, the student is encouraged to incorporate the knowledge gained through this process to build a new understanding and appreciation of the material being considered. The use of evaluation as a process, rather than an end point, highlights an important difference between dialectic and didactic learning. In didactic learning, the professor may tell the students how to evaluate a given situation, the student memorizes this approach and, when asked, can recall (or perform) the evaluation as described by the professor. For example, a professor tells a student how to evaluate a patient to determine if the patient has hypertension. This includes a complete description of how to manually determine diastolic and systolic blood pressure, where to record these values in the patient's chart, and what constitutes normal values. The student is told the values determined in the patient are above the set limit, and the patient is considered to have hypertension. Once the process is memorized, the student can recall each step as described. With a small amount of practice, the process can be demonstrated with an acceptable degree of accuracy.

In dialectic teaching, this process is extended to include a completely different teaching approach. Instead of recalling the normal values for systolic and diastolic pressure, the student is expected to question the validity of the testing method and to determine if a more accurate method is available. Additional questions may be raised about the reliability or efficiency of using a manual blood pressure cuff. Finally, the students may question the validity of the normal values that have been provided. Do these values represent a mean of the population? What happens when a majority of individuals in the population have chronic hypertension? Should the normal values be lowered to reflect healthy values instead of population means? Based on answers to these questions, new approaches may be recommended by the student. These types of questions have led to the use of electronic devices for the noninvasive management of blood pressure in hospital patients; it has also resulted in the lowering of what physicians consider normal blood pressure. Without this type of consideration, the medical professional would be destined to repeat errors from the past.

If students are taught the dialectic approach, they learn how to determine a patient's blood pressure and how to critically evaluate a given situation. Altering the parameter being evaluated to plasma cholesterol concentration instead of blood pressure obviously would be impossible for a student taught using the didactic approach; however, the student who learned to question the process can easily adapt.

In addition to the obvious educational advantages of dialectic teaching using TBL, the methodology also provides practical advantages. TBL brings together practical strategies to ensure the effectiveness of small groups working independently in class with high student-faculty ratios (for example, up to 200 to 1 ratio) without losing the benefits of faculty-led small-group instruction (Michaelsen et al., 2002). Maintaining the learning environment of small groups in large classroom settings should help build higher-order thinking skills and allow students to gain insight through each other's learning processes. Michaelsen stated that the use of small groups takes teaching and learning to new levels of educational significance (Michaelsen et al., 2002).

Paul (1995) emphasizes the need to carefully consider how dialectic education is accomplished in the classroom. In the medical field it is important to discern the validity of information; however, it is also important to consider another individual's viewpoint and to test the validity of the viewpoint using reasoned judgment (Paul, 1995). This becomes particularly important when decisions cannot (or should not) be made on available fact alone. As our knowledge of a disease increases, the facts, as reported in the literature, also change. Put another way, fact is often not the same as truth. Each patient's situation is different and may require a unique treatment plan that is not easily discernible based on facts alone. If we neglect the value of dialogical judgment in medical decision making, we will find ourselves unable to function because of inadequate information.

Teaching students to test the validity of the individual's viewpoint based on reason is of greatest importance. Unfortunately, students often do not come prepared to participate in such activities. In most students' background, traditional didactic lectures have resulted in a passive learning approach where statements made by the instructor are accepted without question. Students need to learn and apply the power of reason gained through critical thinking before offering viewpoints and to apply this same approach when evaluating statements made by others. The extent to which a person accomplishes this process defines his or her level of competency in a given field.

Determining the validity of a statement through reasoning requires a variety of approaches including inductive and deductive reasoning skills. Although most students have acquired rudimentary critical thinking skills useful in daily life, they have been encouraged to disregard the same skills in the educational setting.

EVALUATION OF DIDACTIC AND DIALECTIC TEACHING

Didactic instruction is easy to evaluate; however, the results often suggest an over-inflated sense of true knowledge. As mentioned earlier, students who are able to answer fact-based questions are often tempted to assume that they have mastered the topic. This gives a falsely elevated feeling of confidence, suggesting to the naive student that he or she has the insight needed to apply the information in a real-world setting. This can result in a falsely inflated formative evaluation for the student and/or a falsely elevated summative evaluation. In either case, the student will be misled into believing he or she can perform well in a real-world setting. If the professor (or institution) believes student performance on fact-based multiple-choice tests predicts performance in clinics, both will be disappointed.

The evaluation of dialectic teaching is much more difficult but provides a much greater insight into the student's ability to perform in a real-world setting. This evaluation requires a shift in methodology from a fact-based exam to an evaluation that measures process instead of content. If the goal of dialectic teaching is to produce students who can think independently, evaluations should measure these same skills. In their original 1956 publication Bloom, Engelhart, Furst, Hill, and Krathwohl noted that educational objectives (also called behavioral objectives) evaluate the *product* of the cognitive process and not the *process* that produced the outcome. Objectives written using Bloom and others' taxonomy will be found inadequate in attempting to evaluate the process. New goal and objective statements should be developed that focus on the students' ability to improve their thinking skills. Methods of questioning must also be developed to determine if this has occurred. Standard multiple-choice questions (even second- and third-order questions) will most likely be found lacking.

Evaluating dialectic versus didactic instruction is analogous to judging a diving competition as compared to a 100-yard dash. In diving, judges evaluate the process used to accomplish the dive, not the elapsed time from the platform to the water. Conversely, in the 100-meter dash, no points are awarded for style, and simply measuring the length of time between the starting gun and the finish line chooses the winner. Obviously the latter is easier.

TBL provides an excellent built-in opportunity for the student and instructor to evaluate the dialectic process. One of the most powerful tools is the discussion phase. The discussion accomplishes two distinct evaluation goals. First, it provides a formative evaluation tool for the student. Each student in the group can compare his or her level of understanding to the level of expertise that is expected. Second, it provides the professor with a means of determining the level of performance demonstrated by each student, each group, and the class as a whole.

Discussion, unlike any other form of evaluation, reveals the level of true knowledge and of application skills possessed. As mentioned earlier, Socrates used this approach to extract information from his students while also stimulating individuals to reveal the process used to formulate their thoughts. When individuals initiate a discussion, they will display their level of content knowledge and will also reveal the process used to relate the content to the problem being discussed. This dynamic evaluation process goes far beyond what could be accomplished on a multiple-choice test, or even an essay test. It is difficult, if not impossible, to assess thought process using multiple-choice tests. Essay tests can evaluate the process more accurately; however, this provides students with a starting point that may be above or below their knowledge base. It may also ask them to perform a thought process level that is above or below their ability. Evaluating students' performance through a discussion format circumvents both problems, freeing the students to start at their own level of content knowledge and apply this knowledge using the processing skills equal to their ability. The professor is left with the task of appropriately selecting the case presentation to encompass the content material to be covered and the level of competency possessed by the students. For example, it would be pointless to ask beginning students to diagnose a complex case using data they did not understand, or to process the data at a level requiring skills beyond their training. It would also be pointless to ask advanced students to evaluate a simple case. In either situation, the students will not be challenged appropriately and will not be able to demonstrate their level of skill.

SUMMARY

Didactic teaching transfers content information while dialectic teaching allows students to learn thought processes. Didactic is teacher focused, while dialectic is student focused. Didactic teaching is easy to evaluate, but the evaluation provides little information about the student's thought processes. Dialectic is more difficult to evaluate, but the results of the evaluation process can truly describe the student's ability to process the data and apply it in a meaningful manner in a real-world setting.

TBL is a dialectic methodology that provides an excellent opportunity to teach and evaluate the students' ability to apply knowledge in a meaningful manner. Additionally, TBL allows the dialectic process to be accomplished in a manner that demands group interaction and fosters interpersonal skills, mutual respect, and communication skills. It allows this to develop in a cost-effective manner requiring a relatively small amount of professor time. Learning is focused on the student rather than the professor. When intermingled with other learning experiences, TBL is a powerful tool useful in the medical school curriculum.

REFERENCES

Axtelle, G. E., & Burnett, J. R. (1970). Dewey on education and schooling. In J. A. Boydston, (Ed.), *Guide to the works of John Dewey* (pp. 257–305). Carbondale: Southern Illinois University Press.

Barnhart, C. L. (Ed.). (1872). *The world book dictionary*. Chicago: Doubleday.

Bloom, B. S., Engelhart, M. D., Furst, E. J., Hill, W. H., & Krathwohl, D. R. (1956). *Taxonomy of educational objectives. Handbook I: Cognitive domain*. New York: David McKay.

Dewey J. (2002). Democracy and education: An introduction to the philosophy of education. In S. J. Maxcy (Ed.), *John Dewey and American education*. Bristol, UK: Thoemmes Press.

Flexner A. (1910). *Medical education in the United States and Canada*. Bulletin number four. New York: The Carnegie Foundation.

Kant, I. (2003). *Critique of pure reason* (N. K. Smith & H. Caygill, Trans.). London: Palgrave Macmillan. (Original work published 1781). Retrieved from http://www.palgrave.com/products/title.aspx?is＝1403911959

Liaison Committee on Medical Education. (2007, February). LCME Accreditation Standards. Retrieved from http://www.lcme.org/functionsnarrative.htm#structure

Lujan, H. L., & DiCarlo, S. E. (2006). Too much teaching, not enough learning: What is the solution? *Advances in Physiology Education, 30*, 17–22.

Mannion, J. (2002). *The everything philosophy book.* Avon, MA: Adams Media.

McKeachie, W. J. (1986). *Teaching tips: A guidebook for the beginning college teacher* (8th ed.). Lexington, MA: Heath.

Michaelsen, L. K., Knight, A. B., & Fink, L. D. (2002). *Team-based learning: A transformative use of small groups.* London: Praeger.

Paul, R. W. (1995). *Critical thinking.* Santa Rosa, CA: Foundation for critical thinking.

Pollio, H. R. (1984). *What students think about and do in college lecture classes.* Teaching Learning Issues No. 53. Knoxville: University of Tennessee, Learning Research Center.

Rickard, H., Rogers, R., Ellis, N. R., & Beidleman, W. (1988). Some retention, but not enough. *Teaching of Psychology, 15,* 151–152.

Taylor, E. J. (Ed.). (1974). *Dorland's medical dictionary.* Philadelphia: Saunders Press.

Verner, C., & Dickinson, G. (1967). The lecture: An analysis and review of research. *Adult Education, 17*(2), 85–90.

CHAPTER 6

Team Formation

Kathryn K. McMahon

Through team-based learning (TBL), students learn how to use the power of the team to enhance their learning. It teaches the value of *teamwork* for their future as health care professionals. But teamwork does not just happen—great thought and effort must be made by the instructor to develop and maintain teams so that they work efficiently and effectively. Formation of teams is one of the most important first steps in getting TBL to work in your class.

So what do we want the team to be and how does the formation of the team affect this? We want each team to be a well-working unit that is capable of going through the exercises in an efficient and successful manner and that allows all within the team to learn, understand, and apply the concepts being studied. We also want all of the teams to be successful. Some teams may perform better than others, but for the most part, the difference in performance between the top-performing and the bottom-performing team should not be great. This is accomplished by making sure that there is good distribution of the resources found in the students: background, experiences, course work, previous training.

THREE METHODS FOR TEAM FORMATION

How one creates the teams depends upon many factors: size of class, goals of the course, how diverse or homogeneous the students are, the values of the profession and the institution. The instructor determines what resources are important to be spread through all the teams. Here are three approaches to team formation based upon what is considered most important for resource distribution. The two most important things to do with team formation are (a) don't allow them to pick, and (b) keep the process transparent.

Making Most Assignments Ahead of the First Class Based on Course Objectives and Knowledge of Demographic Variables

Sample: An undergraduate course in nursing titled Ethics in Practice; 75 students in their senior year

A basic demographic questionnaire is sent to the matriculates before the first class, and the following information is returned: average age is 21, 60 are female, all have had one year of closely supervised inpatient care of patients, some have had previous work experience in the health care field. In addition to all students speaking English, about one-third speak Spanish fluently, and several speak one or another language of southeast Asia. Fifty students identify themselves as Caucasian. About 15 students are parents of young children and 5 students have grown children. The instructor feels strongly that one of the most important learning objectives of the course is for future nurses to recognize that people from different cultural/ethnic/language/racial backgrounds have very different perspectives on what defines ethical behavior and how decisions that involve life and death are affected by the values of these backgrounds. How should the students be assigned to teams?

One approach would be to inform the class at the first session that based upon the demographic information submitted *and* the course objectives, assignments to teams have been made to distribute students who speak a second language fluently and have children. So, the instructor creates 12 teams and assigns at least two students to each team who speak a second language and makes sure each team has at least one student who is a parent. The instructor may consider distributing the male students equally, but it would probably be more important that no more than a couple of male students were in any one team. If, after all the students are sitting with their teams, there is a team that has several African American students, then further distribution could be made. Taking the time ahead of class to assign students to teams and then once in the class making the final distribution based on very clearly stated criteria will reassure students that the assignments have not been arbitrary or based on factors not important to their learning the most about ethical decision making. A good Application Exercise question later in the course could ask about the influence of a cultural/ethnic/language background upon the ethical decision-making process; the whole class would have had a unique set of experiences just from the TBL during the course.

Using a Random Approach to Assignment

Sample: A year-long course on pathophysiology for medical students; 100 students, about one-half female

A medical school instructor knows that most matriculates are highly qualified academically, many have had research, EMT, hospital, or other health-related experiences, and most are recent graduates of college. It would be highly cumbersome to identify any particular variable or set of variables that could make a substantial difference in how any one of the resultant 16 teams will perform in this particular subject matter. Therefore, why not assign teams based on something like the students' geographic location of birth?

With the whole class present on the first day of the class, the instructor would ask for the student born closest to the location of the classroom to come forward. The student, most likely quite embarrassed, would come forward and stand next to the instructor. Then the instructor tells the class to spend the next 10 minutes figuring out who was born where, and line up in sequence around the room. The next 10 minutes are noisy and energized as students discover their place of birth. Then the instructor tells the line of students to count off to 16 and repeat, informing them that the number they cite is their team number.

This approach works especially well with a group of students who are just getting to know one another and where the educational atmosphere is one of collaboration and not competition. They love the fate assignments because they ensure that each of the team members is from a different place. It also becomes an important message about the fact that often in life one has to learn how to work with whatever group of individuals one is given.

Distributing a Wealth Item

Sample: A first-year course in biochemistry for veterinary students; 100 students

Since the competition for veterinary school is so stiff, many aspiring veterinarians acquire advanced degrees (master's, doctorate) in one or another disciplines, such as biochemistry, anatomy, genetics, toxicology, or physiology, in order to improve their chances of getting accepted. For a rigorous course in biochemistry that uses TBL as its strategy, it would be important to make sure that students with advanced degrees in biochemistry are equally distributed to the teams across the class. Therefore, at the first class, the instructor could cull those with advanced degrees and distribute them to the teams created by random assignment as described above. Again, keeping the reasoning for this process entirely transparent to all students will help ensure that the students buy in to the fact that the teams were created fairly.

DEVELOPING A GROUP OF PEOPLE INTO A TEAM

Now that the students have been distributed into teams, have you really formed teams? I would argue that you are only halfway there. The formation of a team really is not just the assignment. At that first class, an important and evolutionary process will begin as the students assess one another's personality and approach to working with others. Shy and reticent students will not know whether they can endure those students who are more forward. Those who are more outspoken may think that they will just continue to lead and direct as they always have done. But, in a very short time, especially after feedback on Readiness Assurance Tests and some sharing of feedback on teamwork within the team, all begin to make changes.

It is generally agreed that it takes at least four to five, if not more, working sessions for a small group of people to evolve into a team. Of course, what is happening during this evolution is that the team members are getting to know each other. They are learning that each member of the team, if he or she works at it, can bring important insights, ideas, and solutions to bear on the problems the team must solve to be successful. This is rarely a conscious process in any team member.

Some instructors may feel the need to offer instruction in teamwork, or describe how teams generally evolve (forming, storming, norming, etc. [Tuckman, 1965]), but it is my experience that this is not necessary. Because of the strategy, with its incentives for collaboration and accountability, students learn more about teamwork than what could ever be taught. If you don't believe this, then when you do try TBL, sit down with a team or two after the class gets going and ask what they have learned about working with each other, and what they see as the value of working this way. Even early in a course, they have caught on and appreciate the process. The longer they work together as teams, however, the more robust their enthusiasm will be.

What will best help transform a group of students into a powerful learning team? The team must be challenged at an intellectual level that fosters their collaboration. If the exercises are too simple, the team does not need to work together to be successful. If the exercises are too difficult, even though the team attempts to work together, they will become demoralized and claim that you are not teaching.

Another important issue for the evolution of the team is timely feedback. As teams are just forming, it is very important that the instructor gives feedback on how well the team is performing. The strategy, when followed, ensures this since feedback episodes should occur several times during a TBL session. Also of note, the instructor should know how well the students are learning at several points during the TBL session—something that cannot happen during a lecture.

REFERENCE

Tuckman, B. (1965). Developmental sequence in small groups. *Psychological Bulletin, 63,* 384–399.

CHAPTER 7

Team Maintenance

John W. Pelley and Kathryn K. McMahon

Teams are better at problem solving than individuals for a simple reason. People are complex. This complexity causes individuals to perceive and to process the same information differently, resulting in differing opinions about the same problem. When teams of people are able to compare their perceptions and their decision making in a problem-solving dialogue, they develop a synergy that maximizes the likelihood of a correct decision. A variety of factors can be influential in the development and maintenance of optimal teams. This chapter will first describe a model of the problem-solving process to illustrate how students can contribute differently. Then we will demonstrate how the unique characteristics of groups influence the implementation of team-based learning (TBL). The remainder of the chapter will outline suggestions for individualizing team maintenance in your institution.

THE PROBLEM-SOLVING PROCESS AND THE ROLE OF HETEROGENEITY

After the students have been assigned to teams, a primary goal of TBL is to construct activities that will facilitate team cohesion. Teams appear to be cohesive when all members are actively engaged with each other during the problem-solving exercises. What is not necessarily detectable during this active engagement is whether members have yet developed trust in each other. True team cohesion develops when learners begin to trust each other. They trust not only knowledge of facts, but also each other's ability to apply that knowledge and to apply it effectively. Thus, while factual preparation for the exercise is fundamental and expected, students expect to help each other think about and apply those facts.

Generally speaking, heterogeneous teams will perform better in the long run compared to homogenous teams, because there will be more talent when there is more diversity. However, sometimes it can take a little bit longer for a heterogeneous team to develop the trust necessary to lead to cohesiveness. Nevertheless, it is always better to create a more heterogeneous team because of the advantages in the long run of diversity among teammates.

As described in chapter 6, several methods for achieving heterogeneity sort students based on more tangible descriptors, such as geographical origin or college major. These strategies serve the purpose of preventing students from unconsciously self-sorting into teams of people who think alike because of a common experience or knowledge. However, teams will also have achieved an underlying heterogeneity because of a randomized collection of Myers-Briggs personality types. These personality types represent differences in the way students prefer to process and communicate information, and thus they represent different propensities in the critical thinking process. The Myers-Briggs Type Indicator (Myers, McCaulley, Quenk, & Hammer, 2001) identifies a preference in four areas, described below, to illustrate their contribution to critical thinking. Although these steps are presented in a linear format, the actual critical thinking process should be seen as one of recursive use of earlier steps as appropriate.

CRITICAL THINKING PROCESS

Assessing Data (the Myers-Briggs "Sensing" Preference)

Students problem solve using data or facts. These facts are perceived as a necessary part of the vocabulary in their dialogue. The students prepare for this step in problem solving by reviewing the learning objectives that are provided for a TBL exercise. Clear learning objectives are needed because thinking about the problems provided without the necessary data, or thinking with incorrect data, subverts the rest of the process. More accurate facts and concepts tend to be brought to the group process by those students who prefer (and who have developed) the sensing mental function. They will be seen by their opposites, the intuitive types, as having an enviable capacity to remember facts and details.

Establishing the Possibilities or Solutions (the Myers-Briggs "Intuitive" Preference)

Students use facts to imagine possibilities. Facts help students imagine possibilities because facts are interrelated, that is, they are integrated. This integration helps students to extrapolate from existing patterns and relationships to future patterns and relationships. Thus, integrative knowledge provides a basis for ruling out incorrect answers if the answer choice has clues that don't fit the patterns. The most insightful discussion of the possibilities tends to be brought to the group process by those students who prefer (and who have developed) the Myers-Briggs intuitive mental function. They will be seen by their opposites, the sensing types, as having imagination and a mysterious ability to predict.

Logically Ruling Out the Least Likely Possibilities
(the Myers-Briggs "Thinking" Preference)

Students use logic to decide among possibilities or alternatives. In TBL, those alternatives are the incorrect answers, and a rationale must be developed to rule out incorrect answers. When teams are asked, "Tell us about your thinking," we are asking them primarily about this step in problem solving, that is, the development of a rationale. The orderly process of ruling out wrong answers tends to be accomplished best by those students who prefer (and have developed) the Myers-Briggs thinking mental function. They will be seen by their opposites, the feeling types, as practical and realistic.

Setting a Value on the Solution to the Problem
(the Myers-Briggs "Feeling" Preference)

Ultimately, students evaluate and assess the human impact of the problems and the solutions they choose. They assess the impact on the people involved in the problem and the impact on themselves for having solved it. Human factors contribute to retention of information because emotional involvement in the problem-solving process enhances storage of experiences into long-term memory. Students who prefer the feeling mental function will be most invested when there is an incorporation of human factors in the problem-solving process. Feeling students will be valued by their opposites, the thinking types, for their ability to bring qualitative issues as an additional dimension to their logic.

During this critical thinking process, from evaluating data to imagining possibilities to choosing solutions to setting values, each individual student will have a cognitive preference for one of the four steps over the other three. The cognitive style that is preferred by the individual is referred to in Myers-Briggs theory as the *dominant function*. Thus, when a group has a mix of students with all four dominant functions represented, the group acquires strength in all four stages of problem solving. This acquisition of strength is not limited to the team, since every individual increases his or her abilities in all four steps by engaging in active dialogue. Any student who studies alone is left with strength only in the student's dominant function.

One caveat regarding insights gained from the Myers-Briggs research is that type only indicates a preference for a mental function and does not measure the degree to which the preference is developed as a thinking skill. Just as students of the same intelligence use their intelligence differently and students with the same life or work experience have used that experience differently, so do students of the same type use their type skills differently. Thus, personality typing is best used as a tool *not* to compose teams but rather as a means to help teams understand how each member is contributing and how some misunderstandings might be resolved. Placing the focus on the positive use of learning preferences encourages personal (and thus professional) development instead of creating a stereotypical expectation.

GROUPS AS PROBLEM-SOLVING SYSTEMS—GROUP DYNAMICS

Groups are born as collections, and under the right circumstances develop into teams. Simply bringing people together will not establish a functional team until these individuals learn to trust each other. This is true for families, communities, and TBL teams. After trust is established, the benefits of a team can be realized. In teams in which there is a high level of trust, individuals feel comfortable contributing, engagement is enhanced, and there is a high degree of communication. This clear communication permits the team members to maximize their learning during the problem-solving process since cognitive skills are developed best by hearing and expressing one's thoughts.

It is useful to understand that a group needs time and the proper circumstances until it can evolve from a collection of diverse individuals into a well-functioning team. In fact, it may be counterproductive to expect more from a group than it is capable of achieving in a short period of time. Tuckman (1965) described four stages of group development as (a) forming, (b) storming, (c) norming, and (d) performing. Recognition of the general features of each stage can help educators to better appreciate the limitations of young groups and the process required for groups to become teams.

DEVELOPMENT OF TEAM COHESION

Forming

Group members initially want to be accepted by the rest of the group and to be valued. Initial learning by the team, therefore, includes learning about each other. If a group must solve a high-stakes problem at this stage, group members may spend much of the time thinking about each other rather than the problem. At this stage, a set of rules of operation can help students experience a sense of certainty and security. This allows time to gather impressions and gain experience with each other. This stage can also be facilitated by a training session aimed at creating dialogue concerning roles and expectations. An excellent way of beginning a TBL course is to conduct the first group as a practice session in which TBL is the topic. If the student body is already familiar with TBL, a practice session on another topic is still advisable to help newly formed teams begin to develop. A session in which students are allowed to review previously acquired material is preferable over one introducing new concepts, so that students might have more time for team development in a less stressful environment.

Keep in mind that this first stage in team development is characterized by a desire of each team member to perform by the rules and to be respected for doing that. It might be helpful to let members know that there may be silence and awkwardness, that they might experience anxiety or impatience, that they might test each other or strive for informal leadership, and that all of this is normal and expected. They can also be told to expect that conflict will increase in the next stage: storming.

Storming

The storming stage may be seen as a separate stage, or as the end of the forming stage, since they have common characteristics. The storming stage simply amplifies some of the characteristics of the forming stage. Competition for different roles intensifies. Members are still driven to have respect and certainty in their roles, but as they attempt to organize their efforts they discover the uncomfortable necessity to adapt their attitudes and ideas. The attempt to minimize this discomfort leads to the conflict that characterizes storming. They are frequently conditioned by a culture that promotes memorization and self-advancement. Neither of these skills is necessarily helpful to group problem solving. It is common to hear, "I'm not a group type, I work better alone." Interpretation: "I'm afraid to look dumb, I don't really know what I'm supposed to do or say or how to handle the situation if someone disagrees with me."

During this stage, students may become quite frustrated with group process and not be sure how to resolve conflict. Birmingham and McCord (2004) comment that the use of voting can be quite useful for teams while they are in the storming phase. It is a quick means of ending debate and moving on to the next point. In TBL, it is frequently the case that young teams will use voting early in their development; while more experienced teams will rely on consensus building to come to a decision. If a team becomes stuck in the storming phase, or reenters it, a suggestion to help the development of the team is to use voting as a means of decision making. Ideally, the team will progress in its development where discussion and consensus will be possible.

Norming

The first signs of cohesion are seen at the norming stage. Group members will now have attained an understanding and acceptance of each other and are able to conduct their dialogue in a more positive fashion. Their dialogue will demonstrate more flexibility since the fears concerning loss of respect are gone. Likewise, dialogue will occur with more confidence since individuals will see their roles as valuable and complementary to that of the others. Information and thinking is now shared with high fidelity. Members feel free to debate and they understand that debate can be positive and it can make a positive contribution to learning. This attitude allows students to capitalize on the emotional side effects of debate, namely, long-term memory.

When the norming stage is reached, the teacher can expect a noticeable improvement in the discussion during the group exercises. Rationales will be more numerous and better expressed. It is important to positively reinforce the greater level of discussion at this stage in order to facilitate attainment of the final stage: performing.

Performing

A team that has reached the performing stage has capitalized on the acceptance and trust that characterizes the norming stage and used it to optimize their synergy. Once all members experience the extra benefit of combining different ways of thinking, they are free to continue their development with each TBL experience. The Dreyfus model of acquisition of expert thinking skills (Dreyfus & Dreyfus, 1986) describes this process as a change from context independent behavior (a focus on the rules more than on the situation) to context dependent behavior (a focus on the situation more than on the rules). The acquisition of expert thinking skills is primarily dependent on experience. Thus, the more experience a team acquires in solving TBL problems, the better it tends to perform as a team.

While it is expected that a high-functioning team will eventually reach the norming stage, not all teams will necessarily progress to the performing stage. They may differ with respect to the number of TBL exercises needed, or they may have members who cannot get past the storming stage. It is not essential to the TBL process that all teams reach the performing stage. Teams at the norming stage will work together well enough to achieve the learning benefit that TBL has to offer.

SUGGESTIONS FOR TEAM MAINTENANCE

The overall goal of team maintenance is to help preserve the norming stage and to remove barriers to the performing stage. Based on the theoretical framework given on the problem-solving process, the role of heterogeneity, and group dynamics, the following suggestions may be of value in different health professions education settings.

Schedule Time for Training in the TBL Process

If the TBL method is new to your institution or school, both the students and faculty require training in the method. Indeed, even if the faculty is familiar with TBL, some or all of the students may still need an introduction. Healthy progress through the forming stage requires a thorough introduction to new skills. As an added benefit, faculty who have little experience with the method will benefit from the practice of learning their roles if given practice applications about TBL during the forming stage.

Schedule Time for Training in Peer Assessment

Peer assessment is one of the most controversial aspects of TBL, but it is essential for ensuring individual accountability and preventing social loafing. Students should be oriented regarding the importance of peer evaluation and how it ultimately protects the team and enhances accountability. A variety of different methods of peer evaluation can be used. Whatever method you choose, it is important to orient the teams and explain to them at the beginning of the course what the method will be so that everyone understands how he or she will be evaluated. It is also very helpful to give students an opportunity to have practice in peer evaluation, usually through midcourse formative evaluation.

Another exercise that gives the students practice with peer feedback and can also help them get past the storming stage is: Have the students briefly record on separate index cards a strength that they perceive for each member of the group. Each card is then placed in a stack, allowing each member to collect the contributions of the rest of the team. Members then read their stack to the group and comment on what they have read. The faculty can then ask the groups to react to the exercise and focus on the potential benefits of feedback and its contributions to professional growth. This will naturally lead to a discussion of the peer review system. While this exercise is rather indirect in the respect that it doesn't offer the opportunity for direct criticism of a difficult teammate, it can be very helpful for opening up dialogue about the thorny issue of peer review.

Make Frequent Use of the Phrase "Tell Me About Your Thinking"

An unfortunate habit of novice faculty facilitators is a tendency to prematurely share their knowledge through detailed explanations of the answers to the applications. While explanations eventually have their place in the TBL process, facilitators must wait until the time is right. The TBL process is absolutely dependent on the facilitator asking groups how they arrived at their answer. This process enables other groups to reflect on their interactions, thus providing the feedback necessary to improve their intragroup dynamic. Even if all groups arrive at the same answer, a surprising amount of discussion can result from the backup question, "Did any group have a close second choice?" When the facilitator explores close second choices, groups are prompted to further process differences of opinion that are not discussed when all of the groups agree on the first answer.

Recognize the Need for Adequate Time for Team Development, Including Time Between Meetings for Adequate Preparation

While each TBL course will be different, it is important to keep in mind that teams are not made overnight. Groups must work together for a significant amount of time until they can develop the skills necessary to become high-functioning teams. This does not mean that one cannot conduct brief TBL courses. TBL can even be used in a one- or two-session minicourse. However, high-functioning teams such as are seen in norming or performing teams require significant time to develop, and with TBL courses, this cannot be done quickly because of the need for preparation between sessions. If students are frustrated by a lack of time for preparation between sessions, their contribution to the team will be impaired. Your goal as a TBL course director should be to achieve a balance between time spent providing information to the student for acquisition of new knowledge and then time spent in TBL exercises helping the students learn how to apply the new knowledge.

Consider Other Aspects of Your Curriculum

The maturation and maintenance of your TBL teams will not occur in a vacuum. A variety of influences outside your TBL course can affect the degree to which students are able to accept and embrace TBL. Recognition of these factors is useful when attempting to establish a new TBL course.

1. Where are your TBL sessions located in the curriculum? Early? Late? It can make a difference. Many students are memorization oriented when they enter their health professions training and are accustomed to courses in which passive learning styles are the norm. The intellectual inertia of learning at the memorization level may take more effort to overcome if your TBL course is situated early in the curriculum. In addition, in the early part of the health care curriculum the students' background is more heterogeneous and they are experiencing the stress of rapid adaptation to a new type of education that is more demanding and time intensive. Moreover, these features of the early curriculum may prolong the storming stage for novice students compared with those who have more experience. However, an awareness of this possibility may allow faculty to develop relevant strategies in the forming stage that can mitigate these problems.
2. What type of curriculum do you have? Traditional lectures? Case-based exercises? Hybrid problem-based learning? Many curricula are already evolving in an attempt to organize lecture content around unifying cases so that teaching can have an integrative impact on learning. Other curricula are simply reorganizing lectures in order to better coordinate topics and systems. If unifying cases are in use, an advantage can be gained by coordination with the TBL exercises. If cases are not being used, then TBL might provide a perfect avenue for their introduction into the curriculum.
3. What courses are running concurrently with your TBL course? It is important to be sensitive to the preparation demands of the TBL courses and be aware of what demands might be being made at the same time in other courses. Students are very sensitive to being required to do "too much" reading, or being given Readiness Assurance Tests (RATs) that are either too difficult or too frequent. This can

be especially problematic if there are demanding courses running concurrently with the TBL course, or more than one TBL course occurring at the same time.

These and other questions unique to your own institution may affect the topics and level of intensity you choose for TBL exercises and determine whether the students regard them as an advantage or a disadvantage. The students will see TBL exercises as especially useful if they are perceived as preparation for other course examinations, for the United States Medical Licensing Examination Step 1 (or similar board exams), or for their later use in the clinical setting.

Don't Neglect Opportunities to Reinforce Integrative Learning

One of the many advantages of TBL is that the higher-order cognitive skills teams employ when solving TBL applications can also help students become more effective learners when studying alone. This is especially true for those linear learners (the Myers-Briggs sensing types), who are not as strong in integrative skills. The integration of knowledge is a repetitive theme that underlies many rationales presented by the TBL groups as they defend their answers. If you make it a practice to wrap up each question with your views before proceeding to the next one, you have an opportunity to illustrate what students can look for during their individual study. Since they will have just discussed the question in depth it can serve as a lasting example of how knowledge can be integrated and applied during higher-order problem solving.

Integrative study can be further encouraged in linear learners by overtly demonstrating and discussing the advantages of performing a preliminary overview of new material with an eye to how topics are organized and how concepts are grouped. Integrative study will also provide an opportunity to reinforce in the students the advantage of a self-directed approach to seeking patterns and relationships in their reading as opposed to passively waiting for a teacher to tell them about content.

Give Feedback on Performance to Motivate Individuals and Maintain Team Cohesiveness

In *Team-Based Learning: A Transformative Use of Small Groups in College Teaching* (Michaelsen, Knight, & Fink, 2004), Birmingham and McCord (2004) promote team development by providing tasks that require combining team members' input, that are at the proper level of difficulty (too difficult for individuals but challenging for the group), and that have some inherent interest to the students. They also emphasize the importance of effective reward and performance feedback systems in the development and maintenance of learning teams. Receiving timely feedback on performance, that is, peer and instructor's evaluation of the team's work, is vital to enhancing knowledge of the session's content as well as reinforcing team cohesion and maintenance The advantage of the recently developed Immediate Feedback-Assessment Technique (IF-AT) forms is that they provide immediate feedback to the teams regarding their performance on the RATs. Team development is effected most when the feedback comes soon after the team has performed the task at hand.

REFERENCES

Birmingham, C., & McCord, M. (2004). Group process research: Implications for using learning groups. In L. K. Michaelsen, A. B. Knight, & L. D. Fink (Eds.), *Team-based learning: A transformative use of small groups in college teaching* (pp. 73–93). Sterling, VA: Stylus Publishing.

Dreyfus, H. L., & Dreyfus, S. E. (1986). *Mind over machine: The power of human intuition and expertise in the era of the computer.* New York: Free Press.

Michaelsen, L. K., Knight, A. B., & Fink, L. D. (2004). *Team-based learning: A transformative use of small groups in college teaching.* Sterling, VA: Stylus Publishing.

Myers, I. B., McCaulley, M. H., Quenk, N. L., & Hammer, A. L. (2001). *MBTI manual: A guide to the development and use of the Myers-Briggs Type Indicator* (3rd ed.). Palo Alto, CA: Consulting Psychologists Press.

Tuckman, B. (1965). Developmental sequence in small groups. *Psychological Bulletin, 63,* 384–399.

CHAPTER 8

Facilitator Skills

John W. Pelley and Kathryn K. McMahon

A variety of skills are needed to effectively organize and conduct a team-based learning (TBL) activity. For a teacher who is accustomed to instructing through conventional lectures, it may take some time to become comfortable with the different role required of a TBL facilitator. In contrast to a lecturer, who synthesizes and delivers expert content, the TBL facilitator guides and encourages students to articulate their understanding of the presented problems. Ultimately, the TBL facilitator shares his or her own views of the applications or problems presented to the students. The opportunity to serve as a content expert contrasts with the role of a problem-based learning facilitator, whose primary responsibility is to serve as a guide for the students in their quest to dissect, research, and solve a complex problem. This chapter will review some of the skills that will help instructors to maximize their effectiveness facilitating a TBL exercise.

While the mechanics of running a TBL exercise are important to master so that the process proceeds smoothly, the most important skill for a facilitator is the ability to help teams verbalize their rationales during the large-group discussions. The sophistication of these rationales is often a function of the stage of development the teams have reached. The scenarios listed below pertain to the "norming" (Tuckman, 1965) stage in which students have achieved cohesion and are working together productively. Also included are some discussion techniques for helping students become comfortable speaking in front of the whole class.

TBL SCENARIOS

"Tell Me About Your Thinking."

When groups have either revealed their answers by visible display or by completion of an Immediate Feedback-Assessment Technique (IF-AT) form (a group Readiness Assurance Test), they are ready to explain their thinking. The simultaneous reporting of the various teams provides the richest starting point because the display of answers is their first feedback on how their thinking compares with others. A simple and direct strategy is to begin with any group and ask the group members about the thinking that led them to agree on their answer. Alternatively, the facilitator could ask a team to volunteer to begin the discussion. The instructor should avoid verbal or physical cues that indicate a value judgment on the answer. Facial expression, tonal inflection, or any posture by the instructor that would indicate agreement or disagreement is likely to limit further productive discussion, so the instructor should try to remain as neutral as possible. If the instructor is too positive, any teams that might have offered an alternative rationale might be reluctant to speak in order to avoid embarrassment. This is not as much a problem with IF-AT forms, since the teams will already have been informed whether they got the answer correct. In this case, the discussion can concern lines of reasoning that led them to pick the wrong answer, or it can allow teams a chance to argue for an alternative answer. Be prepared for some surprisingly sophisticated rationales!

It is worth noting that this simple phrase, "Tell me about your thinking," quickly focuses on a team's logic and therefore is a very useful statement for TBL facilitators. A word of caution though—this statement is easy to forget in the heat of the moment when the conversation becomes interesting. Any teacher who is accustomed to lecturing will find out that it takes a great deal of effort to resist offering the expert opinion and continue to ask for the students' line of reasoning. One of the most common errors of novice TBL facilitators is to end discussion too soon to share the answer to the application before sufficient discussion has been elicited. Unfortunately, students will often reinforce a facilitator for doing this by stopping the discussion and waiting for the answer.

"Did Anyone Have a Close Second Choice?"

If every team reveals the same answer, it might discourage you from pursuing the question further under the assumption that all teams thought about the problem the same way. If you persist with an inquiry about their deliberations and the thinking that went into eliminating alternative answers, you can uncover a wealth of analytic thinking that you can reinforce or redirect. Often you will discover that even in a team that chose the dominant choice, there were dissenting opinions. Asking for alternative choices gives voice to the students who might not have had the majority opinion in their teams and provides opportunity for them to articulate their views.

"What Would Make This Answer Correct?"

After you gain experience with the first two scenarios, you might want to look for opportunities to pursue more in-depth analysis of an application. The best answers for these questions are heavily dependent on the data given in the question stem. Since a change in the data given would present a new set of possible explanations, a different answer choice might be preferred. While the examination of alternative patient data does take more time, it maximizes the utility of a given question.

"Here Was My Thinking"

After you are satisfied that a given question has been thoroughly discussed, it is important to provide the students with an explanation of what the answer or answers are supposed to be. A well-defined closure statement for each question is surprisingly important to many students. This is your opportunity to critically analyze the different options and also to explain or reteach areas that may need reinforcement. On occasion, you may want to wait until the end of a series of applications to provide students the final answers, but it is important that you always let them know what the best answers are for the applications so that they can learn from the experience. The emotional energy generated by struggling with an application can substantially augment the learning involved, and sometimes drawing out the experience can further increase the drama and ultimately have an impact on learning.

DISCUSSION TECHNIQUES

The Longest Distance . . .

When a student is speaking to you, the intuitive reaction is to walk closer to the student. However, if you increase the distance between you and the student by walking away, it will draw the student out and assist others who are trying to hear. You may have to walk behind a team that is distant from the speaker. The result is a naturally increased effort on the part of the students to raise their voice so you can hear them. If you position yourself behind the remaining students then, by default, everyone can hear the student who is speaking. This simple technique may feel awkward at first. But remember you are helping the student to speak not only to you but to the student body. TBL works best when the student is speaking to classmates rather than to you, the instructor.

Another way to ensure that the room is quiet and a speaking student is heard is to have any student who is speaking *stand up*. At first, students will resist standing up, but their doing so will guarantee that everyone can hear and that everyone will be quiet! It is probably most effective to make this one of the ground rules for a TBL session: *Stand up* when you have a question or when you are speaking for your team. Also, teams could find a rotational way to ensure that each member carries this task and gets the experience. Unfortunately, health professions students get very little opportunity as students to practice public speaking. This simple approach is one way to help them add this important component to their professional competencies listing.

"Can Anyone Add to This?"

After the first student has responded with a rationale for the group's choice, it is easier for other students to provide additional information. If you ask students from other groups to contribute further, an intergroup discussion will be more spontane-ous. Students are typically less reluctant to offer their group's thinking than to offer their own individual thinking.

"Hide-and-Seek"

If you notice a team (or student) that you want to draw out but who is not responding to the two strategies described above, then you can simply move in closer during the discussion. Moving closer to a team will allow you to naturally alter your focus (and the focus of the student body) to those who might be hiding in the corner.

The different scenarios and techniques described here illustrate some basic differ-ences from a lecture. During a lecture, most of the time is devoted to presenting, organizing, explaining, and illustrating. Lecturing is typically conducted from a speaking platform or stage, and classrooms are not usually conducive to moving among the students. When dialogue does occur, it is usually truncated with affirma-tion from the teacher followed by further explanation. Even interactive lectures rarely reveal how a student is thinking, except by the way a student phrases a question or by short answers to a lecturer's question. The only way to reveal the cognitive proc-esses of a student is to turn the circumstances around so that the explanation becomes the student's responsibility, not the teacher's. In turning around the responsibilities so that the students provide the explanations, a teacher needs a whole new set of skills in order to maximize the learning experience.

Though the experience of facilitating a TBL activity can be initially daunting for teachers who are accustomed to conventional lectures, over time many former lectur-ers never want to return to the stage. In many ways TBL facilitation is far more enjoyable than lecturing. One can do the same exercise multiple times, and each experience is different because of the different interpretations of the student. Even the best lecture cannot compete with the level of energy and degree of engagement in a good TBL activity. There is nothing more enjoyable than facilitating students who are on the edge of their seats ready to debate the next application.

REFERENCES

Michaelsen, L. (2004). Getting started in team-based learning. In L. K. Michaelsen, A. B. Knight, & L. D. Fink (Eds.), *Team-based learning: A transformative use of small groups in college teaching* (pp. 27–52). Sterling, VA: Stylus.

Tuckman, B. (1965). Developmental sequence in small groups. *Psychological Bulletin, 63*, 384–399.

Chapter 9

Peer Evaluation in Team-Based Learning

Ruth E. Levine

Peer evaluation is an essential component of classic team-based learning (TBL), yet many health science educators have encountered difficulties when attempting to incorporate a peer evaluation program into their TBL curriculum. This chapter will discuss the rationale behind peer evaluation in TBL, several methods that have been used to evaluate peers in health science education, the difficulties faculty have encountered when attempting to implement peer evaluation programs, and potential solutions that can be used to overcome these difficulties.

Peer evaluation is certainly not unique to TBL. Educators and health professionals have used peer evaluations in a variety of settings to assess interpersonal skills, foster insight, and promote professional behavior. The literature concerning peer evaluation in health science education is modest in scope, yet it demonstrates a range of outcomes regarding learner acceptance. Several studies of peer evaluation demonstrate positive correlations with faculty evaluations (Arnold, Willoughby, Calkins, Gammon, & Eberhart, 1981; Sullivan, Hitchcock, & Dunnington, 1999; Van Rosendaal & Jennett, 1994) and written exam performance (Eva, 2001; Cheng & Warren, 2000; Levine et al., 2007; Norcini, 2003; Ramsey et al., 1993). In some settings, learners believed that they benefited from peer evaluation; in others they resisted the process. (Greenbaum & Hoban, 1976; Heylings & Stefani, 1997; Levine et al., 2007; Magzoub, Schmidt, Dolmans, & Abdelhameed, 1998; Ramsey, Carline, Blank, & Wenrich, 1996; Reiter, Eva, Hatala, & Norman, 2002; Thomas, Gebo, & Hellmann, 1999; Van Rosendaal & Jennet, 1992; Vuorinen, Tarkka, & Meretoja, 2000; Wendling & Hoekstra, 2002). Learners who accepted the method believed that the quality of their work improved based on the feedback given (Heylings & Stefani, 1997; Magzoub et al., 1998). In other studies, learners who disliked peer evaluation believed that it interfered with their relationships with fellow learners (Levine et al., 2007; Greenbaum & Hoban, 1976; Van Rosendaal & Jennett, 1992). Ultimately, there is no contradiction here. Peer evaluation at its best has the potential to provide valuable feedback to learners from fellow learners, individuals who in many ways are in the best possible position to provide the feedback. Yet in the wrong environment, where there is insufficient training in how to perform evaluation, or a cultural climate of distrust and high competitiveness, peer evaluation can be seen as more of a threat than a benefit.

In TBL, a central tenet of the method is that learners must be held accountable for individual and group work. Peer evaluation has always been regarded as an essential tool in TBL for reinforcing this individual accountability. It is a key strategy for supporting contributions to the group, and avoiding the kind of social loafing than can sabotage other forms of group work. Moreover, peer evaluation can be used to help students become more effective members of a team. When feedback is offered in the middle of a course, students can use the information to significantly improve their skills. As with the general literature on peer evaluation in the health sciences, what has been published on peer evaluation in TBL suggests mixed acceptability by students in different settings. Michaelsen and Fink (2004) described a sense of "fairness" experienced by students who use peer evaluation in undergraduate courses, particularly when a midcourse evaluation is offered to illustrate the impact of the end-of-semester peer evaluation on the overall course grade. Alternatively, students in a six-week psychiatry clerkship reported dissatisfaction with the same method of peer evaluation, albeit without use of midcourse peer review (Levine et al., 2007). Though a variety of peer evaluation methods can be used, Michaelsen and Fink emphasize that three factors must be in place in order for the evaluation to fulfill the purpose of reinforcing accountability. Whatever method is employed it should be capable of (a) accommodating teams of different sizes, (b) accurately reflecting the work of the team members, and (c) making a significant impact on the course grade. They emphasize that when these factors are in place, students are reassured that their teammates will take the group work seriously, and the risk of social loafing is minimized.

In *Team-Based Learning: A Transformative Use of Small Groups in College Teaching* (Michaelsen, Knight, & Fink, 2004), two basic methods of peer evaluation are described, both of which have been adopted by many of the health science programs using TBL. With both of these strategies, students assess the overall contribution of the other members of the team, resulting in a number that is used in calculating each students' course grade (Michaelsen & Fink, 2004). In Michaelsen's method, the number becomes an independent component of the course grade, and in Fink's method, the number is used as a "percent multiplier" of the group's graded work before the final grade is calculated. Copies of the forms that can be used for these evaluations are included at the end of the chapter, but the following is a summary of the methods including their advantages and disadvantages.

METHOD #1: MICHAELSEN METHOD

In the Michaelsen method (see Appendix 9.A), students are expected to assign teammates a score based upon the extent to which they believe their teammates contributed to the overall team performance. As an example, in a six-person team, 50 points are given to each learner to divide among five teammates, with the expectation that the average score will be 10 with a minimum possible score of 7 and a maximum possible score of 13. Learners are also typically prompted to give qualitative feedback about each teammate. The overall peer evaluation score for each learner comes from the sum of the scores provided by each teammate. What is most distinctive about the Michaelsen method is that learners are *required* to discriminate among their teammates. In other words, it is not permissible for a student to give all of the teammates a 10, at least one teammate must get a score lower than the average and at least one teammate must get a score that is higher than the average. This requirement sometimes leads to considerable consternation among learners, especially those who are in high-functioning teams. Frequently students will attempt to "game the system" by making arrangements prior to score assignment that equally allocate the high and low points so that everyone ends up with the same score. Michaelsen believes that this type of gaming should be allowed and not discouraged, *but only if it is done at the end of a term and not the beginning.* If gaming is done at the end of a term, it is evidence that the team is high functioning, and its members probably all deserve to have the same score. However, if students make the arrangement to game the system at the beginning of the term, it is an invitation for some students who have the predisposition to engage in social loafing.

Although Michaelsen has been using this method in undergraduate education for over 20 years with considerable success, a number of health science educators have encountered difficulty when attempting to use this particular peer evaluation process. Medical students in a psychiatry clerkship, for example, complained in their evaluations about the necessity of having to give a teammate a lower than average grade when "everyone seemed good" (Levine et al., 2007, p. 21–22). Anecdotal reports from other medical student educators suggested similar experiences, with dissatisfaction expressed from medical students expected to give any type of negative grade to a peer. This was true in long courses and short ones, but was particularly the case in shorter courses in which there was no midcourse evaluation. Some health science educators abandoned this peer evaluation strategy after experiencing resistance from their learners, while others switched from this form of evaluation to ones in which feedback was mostly qualitative, or evaluation did not count as part of the grade. One can only speculate why the health science educators had more difficulty with this form of evaluation than did Michaelsen with his undergraduate business students. One could hypothesize that the health science students (largely medical students) were more competitive and less compliant than the undergraduates, though this is only speculative. Some students in a conference panel pointed out that they had to live with their fellow students for four years and had to face them in other courses and on the wards, so the risks of giving a poor peer evaluation grade (e.g., less than 10) were greater than if they were just in an undergraduate course together. Another possible explanation had to do with the fact that many of the medical student courses were shorter than the undergraduate courses and did not use the midcourse feedback that enabled the students to become more comfortable with the process of peer evaluation. Nevertheless, even some of the schools that used TBL for an entire year, such as Boonshoft School of Medicine at Wright State University in Dayton, Ohio, abandoned this method because of student discontent.

METHOD #2: FINK METHOD

In the Fink method (see Appendix 9.B), learners are given 100 points and prompted to divide them among their teammates based on the degree to which each teammate contributed to the group work. All members of the team get a "peer score," which is the sum of the points they are granted from each teammate, and then this score is multiplied by their mean group Readiness Assurance Test score (or another group score) to come up with an adjusted group score. In this respect the score is used as a percent multiplier. Learners are also prompted to provide qualitative feedback or reasons for giving the number of points they assigned. In the Fink method, most team members get a score close to 100 points, with those who contributed more getting scores slightly over 100, and those who contributed less getting scores somewhat under 100. Therefore their grade is adjusted upward or downward based on their peer evaluation score. Students generally see this as fair because they can give everyone the same score if they all contributed to the same degree, or they can give different scores if some teammates contributed more than others.

Students take this method very seriously, since it is obvious that the peer evaluation can have a significant impact on the overall grade. Compared to the Michaelsen method, there is generally more satisfaction among medical students, since they have the option of giving all their teammates the same grade if they so wish. A potential problem with this method is that sometimes students underestimate the degree to which they can affect a teammate's final grade with relatively small changes in the peer evaluation scores. This occurs even when the information is clearly provided at the beginning of the course and is illustrated in the course syllabus. As a remedy to this problem, Michaelsen and Fink recommend having teams do a midcourse peer evaluation (Michaelsen & Fink, 2004). The advantage of this practice is it that it not only clarifies the weight of the peer evaluation and gives teams practice with the peer review process, but it also provides valuable feedback for students who may need help with their interpersonal communication skills. Students who are surprised by low peer evaluation scores are particularly benefited by this process, since it gives them the time and the motivation to seek out resources to improve their skills.

Another practice recommended by Michaelsen and Fink to assist with the team process and prevent a difficult end-of-course peer evaluation experience is an analysis and review of the team process about a third of the way through the course. To accomplish this, they recommend a three-step activity. In the first step, students individually identify the behaviors of team members who are helping the team, and behaviors they think members could do to improve team performance. They then share what they wrote with their teammates and rank the top items in each category. Finally, they come up with a list of criteria they think should be used for end-of-course peer evaluation. The advantage of this experience is that it alerts team members to the behaviors that are facilitating or harming the team process without creating the hard feelings that a peer review experience might engender. However, because the review of the team process is an indirect analysis of an individual's particular contribution, some students who are not sensitive might not necessarily perceive if they are engaging in behaviors that are bothersome to their teammates.

METHOD #3: COMBINATION OF THE
MICHAELSEN AND FINK METHODS

Lindsay Davidson at Queens University in Kingston, Ontario, Canada, uses a modified peer evaluation system based on the Michaelsen method. However, the resulting number is then turned into a percentage (e.g., in a team of eight students a score of 73/70 would be 104% and 67/70 would be 95.7%). Similar to the Fink method, the score is then used as a percent multiplier to modify the student's final score. As an example, a student with an unadjusted class grade of 85 who receives a peer evaluation score of 73/70 (104%) would have his or her class grade adjusted upward to 88.4 (85 × 1.04 = 88.4).

As with some other health science educators, Davidson encountered considerable dissatisfaction from her medical students when confronted with the possibility of grade lowering secondary to peer evaluation. She described this dissatisfaction as "bordering on strife and revolt" (personal communication). To address this problem, and still salvage the process, she modified the system so that students with peer evaluations of less than 100% would not be penalized, however, they would still be advised of their scores. Only students who had scores above 100% would have their grades adjusted upward. All students continue to receive composite, de-identified narrative feedback based on their peer's comments.

Following this modification, satisfaction with the process improved considerably. When students asked what to do if they truly felt "everyone was equal," Davidson suggested they assign the 9s and 11s randomly and note it in the comments section. Some groups did this and others worked out how to act in concert with other team members to engineer scores of 100% for everyone. (e.g., gaming the system). In the most recent application of this system, peer scores ranged from 90% to 109% and about 40% of the class received raised grades because of the score.

METHOD #4: KOLES METHOD

Paul Koles of the Boonshoft School of Medicine at Wright State University developed a form currently being used by the teams who participate in the year-long TBL curriculum in the second year of medical school (see Appendix 9.C). The advantages of this form is that it is much more detailed in its quantitative section, asking students to rate their peers in three areas (cooperative learning skills, self-directed learning, and interpersonal skills). Each student is rated in nine areas as meeting a particular competency: never, sometimes, often, or always. Examples include skills such as, "Asks useful or probing questions," and "Shows care and concern for others." Students are also required to complete a qualitative assessment, providing at least one sentence for each teammate to the questions (a) "What is the single most valuable contribution this person makes to your team?" and (b) "What is the single most important thing this person could do to more effectively help your team?" Students must complete the quantitative and qualitative sections on all of their teammates to receive their own peer evaluation score.

Because students stay with their teams for the entire year, they have an opportunity midyear for formative, nongraded evaluation, occurring about five months after the teams are created. The summative evaluations, occurring after 18–20 modules, are worth 10% of the final grade, but the qualitative evaluation tends to be the most useful, since the quantitative scores tend to be typically high and generally do not negatively affect the grades of the persons being evaluated.

This evaluation illustrates one of the disadvantages of peer evaluation when students are *not* required to discriminate, or not given a limit on the number of points to distribute among their teammates. This process lends itself to grade inflation, so that nearly everyone is given a high score. While student satisfaction with this form of evaluation is generally positive, the validity as a grade component is weak, given the universally high scores. Nevertheless, the qualitative component can be quite valuable for professional development.

METHOD #5: TEXAS TECH METHOD

Kitty McMahon and her colleagues at Texas Tech School of Medicine in Lubbock adapted a Professionalism and Communication Assessment Form from the Association of American Medical Colleges and began using it instead of the Michaelsen method to assess and promote professionalism after initially encountering considerable resistance to peer evaluation. This form (see Appendix 9.D) is similar to the Koles method in that it lists several detailed criteria, twelve in total, on which the students are prompted to rank their teammates. Examples include responsibility/dependability, humility, and preparation for learning activities. Each student is ranked on a 5-point scale in which 1 is too little, 5 is too much, and 3 is considered an ideal score. Comments are required for scores of 1 or 5 but are otherwise optional.

For a two-semester course, students were asked to evaluate their teammates three times in a nine-month period. The first evaluation, performed two months into the course, was formative in nature and not used as part of the grade. The second and third evaluations were performed at the end of each semester and were counted as part of the grade. All the data were collected electronically and fed back to the students.

Similar to the Koles method, this form of evaluation was generally acceptable to the students. Qualitative feedback was brief when it did exist and was generally positive. Also, as with the Koles method, the lack of a requirement to discriminate among teammates seemed to lend itself to grade inflation. It seemed to be part of the student culture to give everyone high grades. In fact some students sent e-mails stating they felt more comfortable being honest during the formative evaluation, since they were concerned about the possibility of the summative evaluation having any negative impact at all, even a small one, on a teammate's grade.

SUMMARY

Clearly the process of administering peer evaluation in health science education is a challenging endeavor. As a review of the methods above indicates, there is no perfect way to conduct peer evaluation; each method brings with it advantages and potential problems. Nevertheless, there are some basic principles that will be useful to keep in mind when establishing a TBL program with a peer evaluation component. These principles include the following:

1. The skill of performing evaluation is not intuitive. It is useful to assume that most of your learners have never been taught how to give feedback. A short written or verbal instruction on how to provide constructive evaluation may prove extremely helpful in allaying your students' fears about the process of giving (and receiving) peer review. At a very minimum, this could be included on your evaluation form. Dean Parmelee at the Boonshoft School of Medicine at Wright State University adapted the Michaelsen form by adding the following "helpful feedback comments" derived from Michaelsen and Schultheiss's (1988) article, "Making Feedback Helpful."

    > Providing Helpful Peer Feedback Comments: When giving feedback, keep in mind the seven characteristics of Helpful Feedback: (1) Descriptive, not evaluative, and is "owned" by the sender; (2) Specific, not general; (3) Honest and sincere; (4) Expressed in terms relevant to the self-perceived needs of the receiver; (5) Timely and in context; (6) Desired by the receiver, not imposed on him or her; (7) Usable, concerned with behavior over which the receiver has control. (p. 113)

2. As with any skill, practice is essential in order to become comfortable with the process. Students need to be able to practice peer review in a safe (e.g., formative) environment before they can easily apply peer review for a grade. In a relatively long course this can easily be accomplished through a midcourse peer review. In a shorter course, a more creative solution might need to be considered, such as the "team process analysis" described by Michaelsen and Fink (2004).
3. In many respects, peer review is best received in an environment in which there is a culture of professionalism and a minimal amount of competition and mistrust. The more courses in a health science center that promote and encourage peer review, the better students will accept it and use it constructively.
4. There are benefits to both quantitative and qualitative evaluations, but if students are not forced to discriminate among their teammates (such as giving out only a set number of points), the quantitative evaluation becomes overinflated. Students are most comfortable giving qualitative feedback, and this might be the least controversial and easiest feedback to begin with for the educator who is reluctant to force a discriminatory evaluation on the students. Nevertheless, a peer evaluation without teeth leaves a small group vulnerable to students who are prone to social loafing.

Every educational environment is different, so the best peer evaluation instrument for one setting might not be well accepted at another institution. It is important to keep in mind that while the process of establishing a peer evaluation system can be frustrating (no one ever got a teaching award for putting together a good peer evalua-tion), ultimately it is an essential tool for reinforcing the individual accountability so vital to the process of TBL. Students *need* peer review to feel comfortable that their teammates are contributing their fair share of the group work. What may be best, in the long run, is for educators to experiment with a variety of different methods until they find one that works best for them in their particular environment.

REFERENCES

Arnold, L., Willoughby, L., Calkins, V., Gammon, L., & Eberhart, G. (1981). Use of peer evaluation in the assessment of medical students. *Journal of Medical Education, 56*, 35–42.

Cheng, W., & Warren, M. (2000). Making a difference: Using peers to assess individual students' contributions to a group project. *Teaching in Higher Education, 5*(2), 243–255.

Eva, K. W. (2001). Assessing tutorial based assessment. *Advances in Health Sciences Education, 6*, 243–257.

Greenbaum, D. S., & Hoban, J. D. (1976). Teaching peer review at Michigan State University. *Journal of Medical Education, 51*, 392–395.

Heylings, D. J., & Stefani, L. A. J. (1997). Peer assessment feedback marking in a large medical anatomy class. *Journal of Medical Education, 31*, 281–286.

Levine, R. E., Kelly, P. A., Karokoc, T., & Haidet, P. (2007). Peer evaluation in a clinical clerkship: Students' attitudes, experiences, and correlations with traditional assessments. *Academic Psychiatry, 31*(1), 19–24.

Magzoub, M. E., Schmidt, H. G., Dolmans, D., & Abdelhameed, A. A. (1998). Assessing students in community settings: The role of peer evaluation. *Advances in Health Sciences Education, 3*, 3–13.

Michaelsen, L. K., & Fink, L. D. (2004). Calculating peer evaluation scores (appendix B). In L. K. Michaelsen, A. B. Knight, & L. D. Fink (Eds.), *Team-based learning: A transformative use of small groups in college teaching* (pp. 241–248). Sterling, VA: Stylus Publishing.

Michaelsen, L. K., Knight, A. B., & Fink, L. D. (2004). *Team-based learning: A transformative use of small groups in college teaching*. Sterling, VA: Stylus Publishing.

Michaelsen, L. K., & Schultheiss, E. E. (1988). Making feedback helpful. *The Organizational Behavior Teaching Review, 13*(1), 109–113.

Norcini, J. J. (2003). Peer assessment of competence. *Journal of Medical Education, 37*, 539–543.

Ramsey, P. G., Carline, J. D., Blank, L. L., & Wenrich, M.D. (1996). Feasibility of hospital-based use of peer ratings to evaluate the performances of practicing physicians. *Academy of Medicine, 71*, 364–370.

Ramsey, P. G., Wenrich, M. D., Carline, J. D., Inui, T. S., Larson, E. B., & LoGerfo, J. P. (1993). Use of peer ratings to evaluate physician performance. *Journal of the American Medical Association, 269*, 1655–1660.

Reiter, H. I., Eva, K. W., Hatala, R. M., & Norman, G. R. (2002). Self and peer assessment in tutorials: Application of a relative-ranking model. *Academy of Medicine, 77*, 1134–1139.

Sullivan, M. E., Hitchcock, M. A., & Dunnington, G. L. (1999). Peer and self-assessment during problem-based tutorials. *American Journal of Surgery, 177*, 266–269.

Thomas, P. A., Gebo, K. A., & Hellmann, D. B. (1999). A pilot study of peer review in residency training. *Journal General Internal Medicine, 14*, 551–554.

Van Rosendaal, G. M., & Jennett, P. A. (1992). Resistance to peer evaluations in an internal medicine residency. *Academic Medicine, 67*(1), 63.

Van Rosendaal, G. M. A., & Jennett, P. A. (1994). Comparing peer and faculty evaluations in an internal medicine residency. *Academic Medicine, 69,* 299–303.

Vuorinen, R., Tarkka, M. T., & Meretoja, R. (2000). Peer evaluation in nurses' professional development: A pilot study to investigate the issues. *Journal of Clinical Nursing, 9,* 273–281.

Wendling, A., & Hoekstra, L. (2002). Interactive peer review: An innovative resident evaluation tool. *Family Medicine, 34*(10), 738–743.

APPENDIX 9.A

Method #1: The Michaelsen Method[1]

Peer evaluation   Name_____ Team #____

Please assign scores that reflect how you really feel about the extent to which the other members of your team contributed to your learning and/or your team's performance. This will be your only opportunity to reward the members of your team who worked hard on your behalf. (*Note: If you give everyone pretty much the same score you will be hurting those who did the most and helping those who did the least.*)

Instructions: In the space below please rate each of the *other* members of your team. Each member's peer evaluation score will be the average of the points they receive from the *other* members of the team. To complete the evaluation you should: 1) List the name of each member of your team in the alphabetical order of their last names and, 2) assign an average of ten points to the other members of your team (Thus, for example, you should assign a total of 50 points in a six-member team; 60 points in a seven-member team; etc.) and 3) differentiate some in your ratings; for example, you must give at least one score of 11 or higher (maximum = 15) and one score of 9 or lower.

Team Members	Scores	Team Members	Scores
1) _____	_____	5) _____	_____
2) _____	_____	6) _____	_____
3) _____	_____	7) _____	_____
4) _____	_____	8) _____	_____

Additional Feedback: In the space below would you also briefly describe your reasons for your highest and lowest ratings. These comments—but not information about who provided them—will be used to provide feedback to students who would like to receive it.

Reason(s) for your highest rating(s). (Use back if necessary.)

---

[1] *Note.* From *Team-Based Learning: A Transformative Use of Small Groups in College Teaching,* p. 266, by L. K. Michaelsen, A. B. Knight, and L. D. Fink, 2004, Sterling, VA: Stylus. Copyright 2002 by Larry K. Michaelsen, Arletta Bauman Knight, and L. Dee Fink. Reprinted with permission.

APPENDIX 9.B

Method #2: Fink Method[1]

Assessment of Contributions of Group Members

At the end of the semester, it is necessary for all members of this class to assess the contributions of each member of the group made to the work of the group. This contribution should presumably reflect your judgment of such things as:

Preparation—Were they prepared when they came to class?
Contribution—Did they contribute productively to group discussion and work?
Respect for other's ideas—Did they encourage others to contribute their ideas?
Flexibility—Were they flexible when disagreements occurred?

It is important that you raise the evaluation of people who truly worked hard for the good of the group and lower the evaluation of those you perceived not to be working as a hard on group tasks. Those who contributed should receive the full worth of the group's grades; those who did not contribute fully should only receive partial credit. Your assessment will be used mathematically to determine the proportion of the group's points that each member receives.

Evaluate the contributions of each person in your group *except yourself*, by distributing 100 points among them. Include comments for each person.
Points

Group #:_____   Points
                                                                     Awarded:

1. Name:_____   _____
Reasons for your evaluation:

2. Name:_____   _____
Reasons for your evaluation:

3. Name:_____   _____
Reasons for your evaluation:

4. Name: _____
Reasons for your evaluation:

5. Name:_____   _____
Reasons for your evaluation:

Your Name:_____   TOTAL: 100 Points

---

[1] *Note.* From *Team-Based Learning: A Transformative Use of Small Groups in College Teaching*, p. 267, by L. K. Michaelsen, A. B. Knight, and L. D. Fink, 2004, Sterling, VA: Stylus. Copyright 2002 by Larry K. Michaelsen, Arletta Bauman Knight, and L. Dee Fink. Reprinted with permission.

APPENDIX 9.C

Method #4: Koles Method[1]

Team-Based Learning
Peer Feedback

Team: _____Colleague you are evaluating: _____
Period of Evaluation:

PART ONE: QUANTITATIVE ASSESSMENT *(CHECK ONE BOX FOR EACH OF THESE 12 AREAS)*

Cooperative Learning Skills:	Never	Sometimes	Often	Always
Arrives on time and remains with team during activities				
Demonstrates a good balance of active listening and participation				
Asks useful or probing questions				
Shares information and personal understanding				
Identifies references with relevant information				

Self-Directed Learning:	Never	Sometimes	Often	Always
Is well prepared for team activities				
Shows appropriate depth of knowledge				
Identifies limits of knowledge				
Shows confidence in areas of understanding				

Interpersonal Skills:	Never	Sometimes	Often	Always
Gives instructive feedback				
Accepts instructive feedback				
Shows care and concern for others				

PART TWO: QUALITATIVE ASSESSMENT *(write at least one sentence for each item)*

1) What is the single most valuable contribution this person makes to your team?

2) What is the single most important thing this person could do to more effectively help your team?

---

[1] Used with permission from Boonshoft School of Medicine at Wright State University.

APPENDIX 9.D

Method #5: Texas Tech Method

TEXAS TECH UNIVERSITY HSC SCHOOL OF MEDICINE

Professionalism and Communication Assessment Form, Page 1

Name_____

Too Little<_____SCALE_____>Too Much

PROMPTNESS/RELIABILITY

1	2	3	4	5
Late—colleagues or instructors kept waiting		Routinely punctual—uses time effectively		Wastes time waiting for others to be "on time"

RESPONSIBILITY/DEPENDABILITY

Lack of accountability, actively avoids responsibility and seeks easy tasks		Has team as clear priority, but can balance own life appropriately		Concerned with performance that other aspects of his/her life are damaged

RESPECT FOR OTHERS/TEAMWORK

Disrespectful of colleagues or instructors		Respectful of others		Respectful of others to the neglect of self-respect (self-regard)

HUMILITY

Arrogant towards others		Understands his/her position, but unpretentious		Humble to a fault

ALTRUISM AND COMPASSION/EMPATHY

Concern for self supersedes concern for others, lack of compassion for others		Perfect balance between concern for self and concern for others, empathetic toward others, perceptive		Concern for others to the detriment of self well-being, over concerned resulting in inability to be objective

COMMITMENT TO COMPETENCE AND EXCELLENCE

Low standards of achievement—strives to just pass		Always seeking additional knowledge and skills—lofty goals toward perfection		Driven to excellence to detriment of self and family

SELF-ASSESSMENT/ASSESSMENT OF OTHERS

Lacks insight—poor judge of others' abilities—consistently overrates own performance		Assesses own and others' performance with objectivity and accuracy		Has a self opinion which is excessive

ACCOUNTABILITY/CONFIDENTIALITY

Cannot be trusted with duties or confidential information about others—publicly discusses others by name		Can be relied on to carry out duties and be trusted with confidential information—reminds others of same		Excessive in policing others

RESPECT FOR OTHERS' AUTONOMY AND BELIEFS/TOLERANCE

Bias against persons with differing beliefs or cultures		Tolerant of others—tries to be nonjudgmental		Concerned with others' personally held beliefs to the determent of self

SENSITIVITY TO OTHERS' AND SOCIETAL NEEDS

Oblivious of the needs of others		An advocate for others—helps others when possible—actively seeks appropriate changes		Overinvolved in issues to the detriment of self, family, and colleague needs

TEXAS TECH UNIVERSITY HSC SCHOOL OF MEDICINE

Professionalism and Communication Assessment Form, Page 2

Name_____

Too Little<_____SCALE_____>Too Much

PREPARATION FOR LEARNING ACTIVITIES

1	2	3	4	5
Unprepared for assignments		Well-prepared for activities, knows answers to questions at level evident of advance preparation		Inordinate preparation for assignments to detriment of self and family

COMMUNICATION/LISTENING SKILLS

Inadequate verbal and nonverbal communication skills to effectively communicate with colleagues or instructors		Listens actively to others, restates for understanding when appropriate		Passively listens—Others control time/pace of discussion

adapted from AAMC

COMMENTS (Comments required for assessments scored 1 or 5)

_____
_____
_____
_____
_____
_____
_____
_____
_____
_____
_____
_____

Date_____

CHAPTER 10

Research and Scholarship

Team-Based Learning in Health Professions Education

Paul Haidet, Virginia Schneider, and Gary M. Onady

Team-based learning (TBL) was developed and refined through a trial-and-error process that spanned more than twenty years. This process was guided by theory and empirical research on small-group dynamics, but many of the individual refinements that are part of the method today grew out of the direct observations and classroom experiences of Larry Michaelsen and the early users of TBL.

There are characteristics of health professions education settings that may represent new ground for the application of TBL (see Table 10.1). For example, few other curricula are as rigidly structured. Medical, nursing, dental, and other health sciences students have few choices regarding content or order of courses. Course material is often divided into short systems-based blocks taught by relatively large groups of clinical faculty who are drawn from multiple departments. Depending on the school, there may also be rules that prescribe what activities can be graded, how and when tests can be given, and what the distribution of grades should be. In graduate and continuing education settings these constraints can become even greater, as course activities are usually not graded; learners have competing demands (such as patient care) for their time; and, because of scheduling and other issues, learners are not always all together in the same session. In addition, whole courses may consist of limited contact time, as in single day-long continuing medical education events.

The existing body of experience with TBL forms an important base to guide its use in health professions education. However, the adoption of TBL in health professions education may not represent a simple application of an innovative technology to a new content area; rather, it may require a degree of flexibility in the way the method is employed, given many unique situational constraints. Such a tension between adherence to the details of TBL on the one hand, and flexibility in its application on the other provides an opportunity for research and scholarly work aimed at developing an understanding of how best to succeed with TBL in health professions education. In this chapter, we will first review published scholarly work that has been done about TBL and its use in health professions education. Next, to make explicit relationships observed in the literature, we present a conceptual model to help guide ongoing and future research about TBL. Finally, we conclude with a case example to

TABLE 10.1
Unique Characteristics of Health Professions Education Settings

Typical Higher Education Classroom Setting	Typical Health Professions Education Setting (includes undergraduate, graduate, and continuing medical education)
Courses taught by one or few instructors	Courses taught by large, loosely aligned groups of faculty
Large (> 40 hours) amount of contact hours with students	Contact hours often limited and significantly less than 40 hours
Courses are graded	Graduate medical education (GME) and continuing medical education (CME) settings often do not assign grades
Learners have their time protected to attend class	Learners often have competing responsibilities that include patient care, scheduling conflicts, and so on
Teacher has time protected for planning and implementing a course	Teachers often have to balance "donated" teaching time with funded mandates, such as clinical work and research
Course instructor often has a large degree of control over the grading structure of the course	Medical schools often have mandated grading structures that dictate the number and timing of tests and the grade distributions that must ensue
Course sizes often < 100 learners	Course sizes often > 100 learners

illustrate how one can create opportunities for scholarly work in his or her own experimentation with the method. We note that while our review is mostly limited to published work, much of the progress to date in implementing TBL in health professions education has occurred as a result of additional processes beyond formal publication. Such processes include individual trial and observation, sharing of course materials and artifacts, and conversations among the community of health sciences educators, and have been facilitated by organizations such as the Team-Based Learning Collaborative.

GROUP PROCESS RESEARCH

In TBL, formation and function of learning groups or teams plays an important role in the learning process. Carolyn Birmingham and Mary McCord (2002) present an extensive review of the literature about group process and the development of

high-performance learning teams. To familiarize medical educators with this literature, we present here a brief overview of key results pertaining to group size and
diversity, and the group maturing process. For a more complete discussion of this
literature, we direct the reader to the original chapter by Birmingham and McCord.
First, group size has an important influence on communication and learning processes. A size of five to seven members is considered ideal. In larger groups, individual
members often do not have the opportunity to participate in the discussion, and this
may present a barrier to the group's developing cohesiveness, and may result in lower
satisfaction. On the other hand, while groups with less than five to seven members
may bond and develop greater cohesiveness, the members may not bring enough
variety or amount of knowledge and skills to the group. This variety of experience
and knowledge is a key ingredient in the effectiveness of the group, because it constitutes the resources that the group can mobilize and use in problem solving, leading
to the learning of its members. In addition, groups with less than five members have
increased susceptibility to being distracted by strong or controlling personalities
within the group.

Another important influence on group learning processes is group member diversity in terms of background, personal experiences, viewpoints, and knowledge. Such
diversity tends to help increase the knowledge, skills, and experiences available to the
group to successfully complete tasks assigned to it. However, to achieve higher levels
of diversity, the teacher needs to form the groups and not rely on student self-
selection, which often results in homogeneous groups with low levels of diversity. In
addition, approximately 40 hours of working together tends to be needed for a
diverse group to know how to use member resources effectively. If groups can work
together long enough to become cohesive, heterogeneous learning groups outperform
homogeneous ones.

Finally, the group maturing process has an important impact on collective and
individual learning. As a group moves through various stages of formation (discussed
below), trust is established through shared experience. The group develops common
goals, and members support and help each other for the benefit of the group. The
unique abilities and resources of each member are recognized, and all resources are
better focused on group tasks. Such a matured group has a greater ability to solve
complex tasks, more so than any of its individual members could achieve on their
own. In TBL, the reward structure contributes to the groups' maturation by fostering
individual and group motivation. Individual accountability promotes preparation, as
well as more and better individual contributions to the group. Group accountability
fosters increased commitment to the team and increased effectiveness of team-
member interaction. If the performance feedback is timely (the more immediate the
better), group processes are enhanced because members can immediately see how their
individual effort and the way they work with each other affects group performance.

TBL RESEARCH AND SCHOLARSHIP IN
HEALTH PROFESSIONS EDUCATION

As of November 2006, fifteen articles focusing on aspects of TBL have been published in the health sciences literature, with another four in press. While the majority

of published articles focus on outcomes of TBL, a few report additional aspects, such as development of measurement tools (O'Malley et al., 2003), dissemination of TBL (Searle et al., 2003; Thompson et al., 2007), or communication patterns inherent in different teaching styles (Kelly et al., 2005). Most of the data used in the published literature were collected in the setting of usual curriculum development and evaluation (Dunaway, 2005; Haidet, O'Malley, & Richards, 2002; Hunt, Haidet, Coverdale, & Richards, 2003; Levine et al., 2004; McInerney & Fink, 2003; Nieder, Parmelee, Stolfi, & Hudes, 2005; Seidel & Richards, 2001; Stringer, 2002; Vasan & DeFouw, 2005). Some of these authors (Levine et al., 2004; McInerney & Fink, 2003; Nieder et al., 2005) constructed comparison groups using historical controls selected from within the established curriculum. One study (Haidet et al., 2004) was conducted as an experiment outside the usual curriculum and used randomization to place students into groups taught by different methods.

This small but rich body of literature is emblematic of the strengths and limitations of health professions education scholarship. Given limited resources, combined with ethical principles that discourage practices such as mandatory student participation in experimental teaching trials, most evaluation and outcomes data emerged through observational studies of field implementations of the method. In considering the collective results of these studies, several patterns of outcomes begin to emerge.

KNOWLEDGE-BASED OUTCOMES

A great deal of interest exists around the question of whether students who have experienced a TBL curriculum can outperform students who have experienced traditional, mostly lecture-based curricula. Because assessments of cognitive aspects of performance beyond knowledge retention (e.g., problem solving, reflective practice, creativity, etc.) are difficult or not routinely measured in health professions education, most of the data that exist come from already established testing and evaluation procedures. This limits the conclusions that can be drawn, because most data report on only the dimension of knowledge acquisition/retention, and do not capture the additional dimensions of learning that anecdotal evidence suggests that TBL promotes.

Nevertheless, the accumulated data suggest the conclusion that students in TBL-based courses learn material at least as well as, and in some cases better than, traditionally taught curricula. In the three studies that compared curricula using significant amounts of TBL activities to historical controls, students in the TBL curriculum performed as well on final exams or standardized tests in one (Nieder, et al., 2005), and outperformed historical controls in two (Levine et al., 2004; McInerney & Fink, 2003). Of these latter two, Levine and colleagues have since shown that the students who did better in the TBL course did not do better than historical controls in two other courses that did not use TBL, further suggesting that the improved standardized test scores were a result of TBL, rather than because of smarter or harder working students (R. Levine, personal communication, April 30, 2007). In addition, Nieder and others' analysis of student performance in an anatomy class showed that while average student performance did not differ from historical cohorts, the variance in exam grades was less and the failure rate was lower for the TBL cohort, suggesting that at-risk learners benefited most from the method. In TBL implementations without a control group, reported outcomes suggest that students performed well on course assessments. In Haidet and others' (2004) randomized trial, the performance was not different between TBL and lecture, however, the curriculum consisted of a single session, and many aspects of TBL such as readiness assurance, assigned grades, peer review, and longitudinal exposure to teams were not included.

CLASSROOM ENGAGEMENT

Given the intrateam/interteam discussion format of TBL application activities and the high levels of energy fostered by principles like simultaneous reporting of team answers, it is not surprising that almost all published accounts of TBL included an assessment of engagement. In all of these assessments, TBL has been shown to foster high levels of engagement between students and teachers, students and peers, and with course materials. These assessments range from simple observations, such as low percentages of students leaving the classroom early despite the session running over time (Haidet et al., 2002), to student self-reports and third-party observations using psychometrically tested instruments (Dunaway, 2005; Haidet, Morgan, O'Malley, Moran, & Richards, 2004; Hunt et al., 2003; Kelly et al., 2005; Levine et al., 2004; Seidel & Richards, 2001; Stringer, 2002; Vasan & DeFouw, 2005). Classroom engagement in these studies is generally defined as students remaining on task, communicating actively with each other and with the teacher and not performing off-task behaviors, such as reading newspapers, checking e-mail, and so forth. In addition, several qualitative course evaluations (Hunt et al., 2003; Levine et al., 2004) have suggested that increased student engagement with course materials in the form of more thorough advance reading and preparatory work, is a primary mechanism leading to enhanced knowledge assessments in TBL-based courses.

Beyond measuring levels of engagement through either quantitative or qualitative methods, there has been little work to illuminate why learners are more engaged. Recent evidence from one study (Levine, Kelly, Karakoc, & Haidet, 2007) suggests that the relationships among students on individual teams and students' perceptions of their contributions to the team's performance were powerful motivators for students to engage with course material and with each other during course sessions.

LEARNER ATTITUDES

Studies performed to date have employed a number of perceptual measures of attitudes about course content, session or course effectiveness, the usefulness of working in teams, and the utility of TBL itself. While most of these studies demonstrated favorable attitudes toward aspects of TBL, not all did, and the collective results of these initial studies paint an interesting and complex picture of TBL from the learner's perspective. Initial observations at Wright State University and elsewhere (Haidet et al., 2002; Seidel & Richards, 2001) showed that students and residents had favorable attitudes toward TBL itself, and that their attitudes toward the content being taught improved after sessions that employed TBL techniques.

Further controlled and uncontrolled studies with undergraduate, graduate, and preclinical medical students echoed these initial favorable attitudes toward TBL (Dunaway, 2005; McInerney & Fink, 2003; Nieder et al., 2005). In addition, Levine and others (2004) demonstrated that clinical medical students' perceptions of the value of learning in teams improved after participating in a TBL course. However, Hunt and others (2003) showed that while students performed desired learning behaviors in a preclinical medical student TBL course in evidence-based medicine, many students devalued the TBL method as inefficient and of limited effectiveness. These results were echoed in the randomized trial (Haidet et al., 2004). Given the limitation that the trial only compared single learning sessions (and groups did not have enough longitudinal time to form properly), it nevertheless found significant differences in student attitudes between the active learning (informed by TBL) and lecture arms. Students in the active learning arm felt that the session was significantly less effective at achieving specified learning goals, and felt that they learned less during the session when compared to students in the lecture arm. These findings exist in the context of those same active learning students perceiving themselves to be (and objectively observed to be) more engaged than the lecture students. In addition, both active learning and lecture-based students achieved the same results on knowledge assessments before and after the sessions. The authors suggested that active learning methods such as TBL may challenge students' basic assumptions about what is effective teaching and may lead to lowered perceptions of the value of such methods, even though students may learn material just as well and are more engaged while doing so. As more educators experiment with TBL in their own teaching, it will be important to continue the study of learner attitudes and begin to assess teacher attitudes in order to better understand how perceptions modify the TBL experience and affect learning outcomes.

A CONCEPTUAL MODEL FOR SCHOLARLY WORK ON TBL IN HEALTH PROFESSIONS EDUCATION

Given the unique characteristics of health professions education and the contextual constraints that such characteristics place on TBL application, there is a need for further scholarship with regard to implementation and evaluation. For example, the communities of educators who use TBL generally agree that a significant amount of contact time (typically about 40 hours) is needed for groups of students to form into high-performance learning teams (Birmingham & McCord, 2002). However, such large amounts of contact time are rarely available to single courses in health sciences curricula. This tension between the ideal and the possible, in terms of contact time, leads to several potential questions for scholarly work:

1. What learning benefits can be expected from TBL courses that have low amounts of team contact time?
2. Can the patterns of interaction characteristic of high-performance learning teams be achieved if student assignments to teams are maintained across courses or rotations?
3. Does the "40 hour rule" hold for all courses or situations? Can groups form into high-performance learning teams more quickly with training or in special contexts, such as the clinical ward environment?
4. Does prior participation in a TBL experience at one point in the curriculum allow for shorter needed duration of contact time to form a high-performance team during courses at later points in the curriculum?
5. Does higher performance of teams translate into increased student learning in the course?

If TBL is to be maximally successful, educators need to pursue these and other areas of inquiry in order to build the knowledge base about the most effective TBL use in health sciences settings.

While the important questions will emerge as educators gain increasing experience with the method, the field itself will benefit if its scholars are working from a common frame of reference. This is where a conceptual model can help, because it can provide a background map of the theory and findings in the field. For TBL, a conceptual map can be drawn based on the generally accepted assumptions, theory, observations, and results that led to the method's development, as well as findings to date from the studies in health sciences education. We present a conceptual model in Figure 10.1. Our goal is to make explicit some of the assumptions about TBL and its effects on learning, and to stimulate the process of brainstorming and formulating questions for scholarly work. We anticipate that the model will change and be modified as data are collected and new conclusions are drawn about the model's elements and relationships.

Learner engagement forms a central concept in the model. A foundational assumption of TBL is that activities that foster students' meaningful engagement with course content and with each other will ultimately lead to favorable learning outcomes. This assumption is at the heart of most educational learning theories (Bransford, Brown, & Cocking, 2000) and has been described in many different forms. For example, Parker Palmer (1998) describes the "Community of Truth" as an ideal learning setting where dialogue between and among learners and teacher fosters a deep engagement with and understanding of the subject of study.

In the conceptual model, we characterize the use of TBL as a series of design decisions that together create a learning environment specifically aimed at fostering

FIGURE 10.1
Conceptual Model for TBL

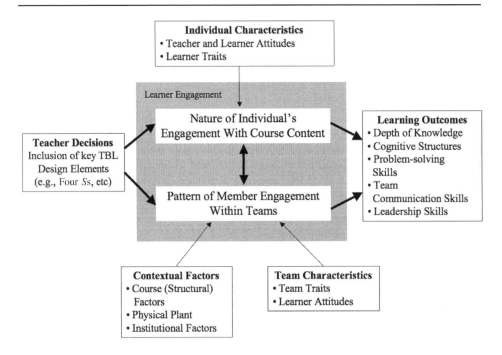

high degrees of learner engagement. This learner engagement exists on two interrelated levels. First is the engagement of individual learners with course content. While this engagement may be represented by individual study and advance preparation, it also implies a deep interaction with the subject as the student ponders, hypothesizes, searches for related information, and connects the course content to knowledge that the student already possesses. In short, engagement with course content implies a process of integration whereby students begin to incorporate course material into their own knowledge, understanding, and experience (Dewey, 1938).

A second form of learner engagement is what happens within the learning teams. The field of group process research has produced several theories of group development that suggest that high-performing teams progress through a number of developmental stages, such as the forming, storming, norming, and performing stages proposed by one of the more well-known theories (Tuckman, 1965). These theories of group development have a significant degree of overlap, and all suggest that a high-performing team can be characterized by patterns of interaction that allow the team to maximally access the unique strengths of its individual members and use these strengths in accomplishing the team's goals.

The central core of the conceptual model, represented by the bold arrows in Figure 10.1, suggests that design decisions by the teacher, such as the decision to format in-class application activities to follow the four Ss, have an impact on the degree and quality of learner engagement, as represented by learners' relationships with course content and each other. Learner engagement with content and within teams is interrelated and potentially mutually reinforcing. For example, in focus groups of core-clerkship psychiatry students who had experienced a TBL curriculum, students overwhelmingly identified a desire to "not let their team down" as the primary motivating factor to pursue individual reading prior to classroom sessions (R. Levine, personal communication, March 3, 2003). Greater degrees of and higher-quality engagement both with content and other learners are expected to favorably affect a variety of learning outcomes, such as knowledge, skills, and attitudes.

The additional boxes in Figure 10.1 acknowledge the influence that mediating factors such as individual and team characteristics and context have on learner engagement. While the model is not intended to portray an exhaustive list of such mediating factors, it is intended to suggest that some factors may be more influential than others either on engagement with course content or engagement within teams. For example, individual characteristics such as teacher enthusiasm for the topic, teacher satisfaction, how much learners value the subject, how much incentive learners have to pursue a good grade in the course, and learners' prior experience and academic abilities may all have an impact on the degree and quality of individual learners' engagement with course content.

In a similar fashion, a number of course-specific and institutional contextual factors, such as the amount and regularity of contact hours during the course, the acoustics and comfort of the classroom, what is simultaneously or sequentially going on in other courses, and the culture of the school toward learning, can all influence the amount and quality of engagement in TBL course activities.

Also, characteristics of teams themselves, such as the mix of personalities on particular teams, leadership within teams, and compatibility in cognitive or emotional styles; and learner attitudes, such as the amount of value placed on working in teams, and learners' definitions of what is good teaching, will all have an impact on the ability of teams to develop patterns of behavior that maximize performance. The presence of mediating factors may modify the success of a particular TBL implementation, and their measurement, where possible, can help educators to better understand the context and plan an approach when adapting TBL to health professions education settings.

The conceptual model is intended to assist TBL scholars by providing a common reference point for formulating questions, developing methods, and designing evaluation strategies. In order to promote the evolution of the field and expand the knowledge base with respect to the details of TBL implementation in health professions settings, educators need to continue to pursue and disseminate scholarly work based on their experiences with the method. In the final section of this chapter, we present a case study intended to illustrate the use of the conceptual model in pursing scholarly work in the setting of one's usual educational activities.

CASE STUDY: AN INTEGRATED COURSE IN A FIRST-YEAR MEDICAL SCHOOL CURRICULUM

The intent of this case study is to empower readers to explore opportunities for scholarly work as they plan TBL implementations. The case is inspired by informal stories of scholarship that surround many of the TBL medical education publications to date. We have organized the case to illustrate possible opportunities based on specific components of the conceptual model. In an actual implementation, we would suggest that educators consider questions germane to their own context, the resources available, and the significance that their findings will have for the field in general. We feel that a key ingredient of successfully completing a scholarly project is for educators to choose a single or limited number of questions. Choosing a single or limited number of related questions will allow the educator to remain focused and on task and will enhance the likelihood of successfully completing and communicating the results of one's TBL experience.

Case Background

The faculty curriculum committee at a midsize (120 students per year) medical school plans to integrate the fall and spring semesters of its first-year curriculum. Four departments, under the guidance of two course directors (one for each semester), will now need to work together toward integrating this new curriculum. Course directors begin to recruit faculty to work on content for the new curriculum. The leadership of the medical school informs the course directors that it wants to increase the amount of "active learning" and reduce the amount of lectures, however, it does not specify what exact methods teachers should use to achieve this. The course directors both agree that, given limited numbers of faculty and protected time for teaching, TBL is a good choice to use for the active learning sessions.

Team Traits

When the TBL faculty begin to design common elements of the course, they wrestle with strategies for assigning students to teams. All of the teachers are in agreement that the course directors should assign the teams (as opposed to students self-selecting teams), but no particular student background information seems pertinent in terms of course content and team assignment. One option would be to randomly assign students to teams; however, some of the faculty with business school experience suggest that a more systematic method of assigning teams might maximize performance.

SCHOLARLY QUESTION: (a) Will a personality- or cognitive-based system for assigning students to teams (e.g., Myers-Briggs), as opposed to random assignment, lead to enhanced team performance?

METHOD: The faculty decides to reshuffle the teams after the first semester, so that they can use both methods (random assignment and a personality-based system) in a single year with the same class. In the first year of doing the course, the course directors will use the personality-based system to assign teams in the first semester, and random assignment in the second semester. In the second year of doing the course, the directors will use random assignment in the first semester, and the personality-based system in the second semester. The faculty will use the same individual Readiness Assurance Tests (IRATs,) group Readiness Assurance Tests (GRATs), and final exams in both years. During the course, the teachers of each session will keep notes about the quality of interactions that they observe within teams during the session. At the end of each year, the faculty will compare these notes between the two semesters within that year. At the end of the two-year cycle, the faculty will compare group-based (e.g., GRAT) and individual-based (e.g., IRAT, final exam) grades between the two years.

Physical Plant

A lab area containing 10 workstations is available; using this space will necessitate 10 teams of 6 students to be distributed among the workstations. Each session would need to be conducted twice, once with each half of the class. Alternatively, a lecture hall that can accommodate the entire class is available. Both spaces are equipped with cameras that will allow videotaping of sessions. As the course directors ponder the decision on which space to reserve (and the extra work that using the smaller space will require), they begin to wonder what effect, if any, the physical layout of the room and the overall class size has on the learning process.

SCHOLARLY QUESTIONS: (a) How does the physical layout of the room affect student interaction in learning teams? (b) Does the overall class size have an impact on the quality of discussion that occurs during whole-class (e.g., interteam) discussions?

METHOD: The course directors decide to conduct the fall semester in the lab space, and the spring semester in the lecture space. Next year, they will reverse the order and conduct the fall semester in the lecture space and the spring semester in the lab space. They arrange for videotaping of all of the TBL sessions, and engage the faculty teaching the sessions to agree to a five-minute interview after each session to comment on the quality of discussion during that session. The course directors plan to review the videotapes to assess the body language of the groups during each session, and as part of their planned faculty development process, engage their faculty to review the tapes and comment on the quality of the facilitation and the quality of the discussion by students. The course directors themselves plan to review all the tapes and comment on any particular patterns of communication that are evident on the tapes. At the end of two years, the course directors plan to review the faculty interview data, the body language data, the faculty videotape review data, and their own videotape reviews to look for systematic differences between patterns of interaction and quality of discussion between the two venues.

Teacher Decisions

During the first year of the course, the teachers use a TBL peer review process that requires each student to evaluate fellow team members. The course directors provide each student with a certain number of points that the student must distribute among the team members. Students are required to differentiate in distributing these points; for example, they cannot give the same number of points to more than two of their team members. The peer review score that each student receives from his or her teammates is then used as part of that student's overall course grade. During the year, the course directors receive a number of complaints from students about the peer review process. A central theme in these complaints seems to be that the students feel that it is unfair to require them to grade their peers, and that some teams are "gaming" the process, meaning that they are prearranging the grades. The course directors begin to wonder how the peer review process is influencing the work of the teams, and whether they should continue to use it in following years.

SCHOLARLY QUESTION: (a) How does the peer review process influence students' actions with regard to advance preparation and interactions within their teams?

METHOD: The faculty decides to pursue a formal qualitative course evaluation with respect to the peer review process. They randomly select 40 students to participate in three focus groups on the topic, assuming that random selection should provide a sample with a balanced mix of student attitudes with regard to peer review (if such a balance exists). In addition, the selection process is structured so that each focus group has no more than one student from any of the given course teams, to ensure that the students feel safe to give honest answers about their team's dynamics during the focus groups.

The course directors secure funding from the dean of education to provide each participating student with a $50 stipend, and they use this stipend to enhance focus group recruitment. The instructors devise a focus group interview guide that contains probes about students' perceptions of (a) the effects of the peer review process on individual students' engagement in the course and (b) the effects of the peer review process on the dynamics of communication within their teams. The directors engage a faculty member with qualitative research expertise who was not involved with the course to moderate the focus groups, and they brief this faculty member on the nature of TBL and the issues involved with peer review. The directors also engage their administrative assistant to transcribe audiotapes (and remove the identity of participants) of the focus group discussion, and they plan to pursue an analysis of these transcripts that is aimed at understanding the meanings that students attach to peer review, and the implications that these meanings have for individual and team engagement.

The three projects outlined here represent a small sample of the rich opportunities for scholarship that exist when implementing TBL in health professions education. We have chosen specific areas of the conceptual model to demonstrate how the model can facilitate brainstorming and exploring options for particular projects. Once opportunities for scholarly work are identified, they can be ordered and compared on (a) feasibility and (b) importance of information gleaned. In this way, administrators, course directors, teachers, and other stakeholders can begin to form a research agenda for their individual institution that is aimed at advancing the best methods of integrating TBL into the medical curriculum.

CONCLUSION

In conclusion, TBL is built on foundations of group process theory and research as well as on the ongoing observations and trials of its pioneers. Health professions education represents a unique and exciting context in which to adapt TBL. The ultimate success of this endeavor will be significantly affected by the scholarly activities of individual health professions educators as they conduct, evaluate, and communicate their own experiences with the method.

REFERENCES

Birmingham, C., & McCord, M. (2002). Group process research: Implications for using learning groups. In L. K. Michaelsen, A. B. Knight, & L. D. Fink (Eds.), *Team-based learning: A transformative use of small groups* (pp. 73–94). Westport, CT: Praeger.

Bransford, J. D., Brown, A. L., & Cocking, R. R. (Eds.). (2000). *How people learn: Brain, mind, experience, and school.* Washington, DC: National Academy Press.

Dewey, J. (1938). *Experience & education.* New York: Touchstone.

Dunaway, G. A. (2005). Adaptation of team learning to an introductory graduate pharmacology course. *Teaching and Learning in Medicine, 17*(1), 56–62.

Haidet, P., Morgan, R. O., O'Malley, K. J., Moran, B. J., & Richards, B. F. (2004). A controlled trial of active versus passive learning strategies in a large group setting. *Advances in Health Sciences Education, 9*(1), 15–27.

Haidet, P., O'Malley, K. J., & Richards, B. F. (2002). An initial experience with team learning in medical education. *Academic Medicine, 77*(1), 40–44.

Hunt, D. P., Haidet, P., Coverdale, J. H., & Richards, B. F. (2003). The effect of using team learning in an evidence-based medicine course for medical students. *Teaching and Learning in Medicine, 1*(2), 131–139.

Kelly, P. A., Haidet, P., Schneider, V., Searle, N., Seidel, C. L., & Richards, B. F. (2005). A comparison of in-class learner engagement across lecture, problem-based learning, and team learning using the STROBE classroom observation tool. *Teaching and Learning in Medicine, 17*(2), 112–118.

Levine, R. E., O'Boyle, M., Haidet, P., Lynn, D., Stone, M. M., Wolf, D. V., & Paniagua, F. A. (2004). Transforming a clinical clerkship through team learning. *Teaching and Learning in Medicine, 16*(3), 270–275.

Levine, R. E., Kelly, P. A., Karakoc, T., & Haidet, P. (2007). Peer evaluation in a clinical clerkship: Students' attitudes, experiences, and correlations with traditional assessments. *Academic Psychiatry, 31*, 19–24.

McInerney, M. J., & Fink, L. D. (2003). Team-based learning enhances long-term retention and critical thinking in an undergraduate microbial physiology course. *Microbiology Education, 4*(1), 3–12.

Nieder, G. L., Parmelee, D. X., Stolfi, A., & Hudes, P. D. (2005). Team-based learning in a medical gross anatomy and embryology course. *Clinical Anatomy, 18*(1), 56–63.

O'Malley, K. J., Moran, B. J., Haidet, P., Seidel, C. L., Schneider, V., Morgan, R. O., Kelly, P. A., & Richards B. F. (2003). Validation of an observation instrument for measuring student engagement in health professions settings. *Evaluation & The Health Professions*, *26*(1), 86–103.

Palmer, P. (1998). *The courage to teach*. San Francisco: Jossey-Bass.

Searle, N. S., Haidet, P., Kelly, P. A., Schneider, V. F., Seidel C. L., & Richards, B. F. (2003). Team learning in medical education: Initial experiences at ten institutions. *Academic Medicine*, *78*(Suppl. 10), 55–58.

Seidel, C. L., & Richards, B. F. (2001). Application of team learning in a medical physiology course. *Academic Medicine*, *76*(5), 533–534.

Stringer, J. L. (2002). Incorporation of active learning strategies into the classroom: What one person can do. *Perspectives on Physician Assistant Education*, *13*(2), 98–102.

Thompson, B. M., Schneider, V. F., Haidet, P., Levine, R., McMahon, K., Perkowski, L., & Richards, B. F. (2007). Team learning at ten medical schools: Two years later. *Medical Education*, *41*, 250–257.

Tuckman, B. W. (1965). Developmental sequence in small groups. *Psychological Bulletin*, *63*(6), 384–399.

Vasan, N. S., & DeFouw, D. (2005). Team learning in a medical gross anatomy course. *Medical Education*, *39*(5), 524.

PART II

Voices of Experience

CHAPTER 11

Team-Based Learning in the Premedical Curriculum

Genetics

Dorothy B. Engle

In 1999, the world braced for the millennium bug, Prince Edward married Sophie Rhys-Jones, and I attended a faculty development workshop on team-based learning (TBL) given by Larry Michaelsen. In my opinion, the most significant of these events was the TBL workshop.

I was in my third year of teaching college-level genetics. Genetics is a required course for biology majors and is highly recommended for all of our preprofessional health students. Genetics is different from most other areas of biology, because it is both a subdiscipline and a technology. As a subdiscipline of biology, genetics focuses on inheritance and the means by which genes, the units of inheritance, cause organisms to display various characteristics. In addition, genetics is also a tool kit composed of strategies that are applicable to almost every area within biology, from biochemistry to physiology to ecology. In this way it is similar to mathematics: once you understand how to approach and solve a certain type of problem, you can apply this knowledge to a wide variety of questions. The exceptional power of genetics as an experimental approach, especially at the molecular level, has made it vitally important to every field of biology as well as to medicine, veterinary science, and law enforcement. As we learn more about the underlying genetic bases for many diseases, it is clear that in the context of preprofessional health education, a thorough foundation in genetic principles and a clear understanding of genetic technology is essential.

WHY I ADOPTED TBL FOR COLLEGE-LEVEL GENETICS

For three years, I taught genetics the "normal" way: I lectured most of the time, with some modeling of problem-solving strategies and a little casual in-class group work. Students did most of the chapter problems on their own or in optional homework clubs. Although they performed as expected, with the usual numbers of high, medium, and low test scores, I was continuously haunted by a vague sense of dissatisfaction. Although most students could recap classic experiments and discuss their significance, few could apply this knowledge to propose experiments addressing a new situation. They became proficient at simple calculation problems using small data sets, but could not string together conclusions from a series of experiments to get a complete story. From the students' perspective, the familiar lecture format was serving them well. As juniors, most of them had already figured out how to get decent grades in biology classes, and those planning to apply to medical school needed only a superficial understanding of genetics for the Medical College Admission Test (in recent years, on the other hand, there are more complex genetics problems on the MCAT, making this course even more important to our premed population). As far as I was concerned, however, something was wrong. I wanted to produce geneticists, but I was getting genetic historians. I knew that it was not their fault but mine. Naturally, the students were blissfully unaware of my growing discomfort.

My other dissatisfaction with the genetics course involved fairly typical student behavior. Although I gave frequent reminders to review old material prior to lecture, diagnostic quizzes showed that the majority of the class failed to do this, so I ended up re-covering the concepts from general biology. (I teach the introductory course myself, so they can't get away with feigning ignorance.) Why should they do the work when I was willing to do it for them? In addition, there was the age-old habit of cramming the night before the test.

In 1999 Larry Michaelsen was invited by the faculty development office to teach us about TBL. I expected to pick up a few teaching tricks at the workshop, but I did not expect to be completely transformed. As Larry outlined the methods and compared the outcomes of lecture only versus TBL, I was stunned. The most profound lesson I learned was that by lecturing most of the time, I was wasting precious class hours doing what students could do on their own. Simultaneously, I was sending them home with work that called for my help and guidance. Concerned about covering content, I spent valuable time explaining simple definitions that could have been easily comprehended from reading the text. Likewise, I was reviewing old material that students should have managed independently. Although I was modeling problem-solving techniques, there was not enough time left in class for significant practice; most of the practice time was out of class. Furthermore, because students are busy, attempts to encourage group work outside of class were unproductive and frustrating. Fortunately, the TBL workshop included much how-to information that I could easily adapt to my particular course. Armed with the Michaelsen model to follow (and a new textbook), I bravely scrapped the entire course and started over. Because genetics is largely about problem solving, it was relatively easy to rework the content into a TBL format.

IMPLEMENTING TBL IN GENETICS

In January 2000 I launched the new and improved genetics course to a skeptical (but not hostile) class. As their first college biology teacher, I had already earned their trust by helping them successfully negotiate the transition from high school. Now two years later, I took shameless advantage of that trust. We followed the basic TBL format: assigned reading, individual Readiness Assurance Tests (IRATs) and group Readiness Assurance Tests (GRATs) and appeals, short clarification of complex ideas, then several class periods of problem solving. I modeled strategies with the whole class, then the teams worked on similar examples while I circulated and eavesdropped. We worked our way up from simple questions to thornier problems, with relevant homework between each class. Most of the problems came from the textbook, although I generated several application scenarios that incorporated content from multiple chapters. Other graded activities included analyzing research articles (individual and group) and a group research proposal.

Prior to TBL, the usual pattern followed by students was to hear a lecture first, then delve into the chapter using the lecture notes as a guide. Thus reading ahead of time to prepare for class was a new but key behavior that I wanted to reinforce. In that first TBL offering, it quickly became apparent that students had trouble focusing on their initial chapter reading. Not surprisingly, they lacked the experience to distinguish important details from trivial details. Without a prior lecture as a guide, some were just skimming and others were trying to memorize every fact. This was easily remedied midstream by the creation of Reading Guides for each chapter. In the Reading Guides, I pointed out what information should be familiar from the first-year introductory course, asked leading questions concerning information they should have gained from the reading, and highlighted what concepts would be further clarified in class. Having answered the questions in the Reading Guide, the students arrived in class with a partial set of notes already written. If a particular chapter was highly challenging, or had all new information, I allowed a brief question-and-answer session before the RATs. Because I am constrained by a 50-minute time period, the RATs were relatively short. I used Scantron test forms for the IRATs; lately we have used Immediate Feedback-Assessment Technique (IF-AT) scratch-off sheets for the GRAT, allowing for instant feedback. The RATs clearly indicated who was prepared for class and who was not. To accommodate excused absences, we dropped the lowest IRAT and GRAT score for the final grade.

The group dynamics were evaluated using a peer evaluation score. This is the one area I have changed the most since the first TBL offering. Initially I counted peer evaluation scores as 10% of the grade, with students assigning points to teammates. For example, in a team of six members, each person would have 50 points to distribute to the five other team members. They were required to assign at least one score of 11 and at least one score of 9. Given my particular population of students, there were two problems with this strategy. First, the forced differential scoring caused much consternation among highly functioning groups in which all the members pulled their weight. Second, I discovered that having one disastrously bad person in a team of six was actually an advantage, as giving the slacker a very low score freed up points to assign to the other teammates. This led to intergroup score disparities among the good students; the best student in a well-functioning group might get 11 points, while an equally talented student in a group with one loafer might earn 15 points. Consequently, I recently changed to a fraction system, in which teammates receive a fraction of the group points according to their participation. In most cases students merit a 1, or all group points earned, with the relatively few slackers getting only some fraction of the group total.

OUTCOMES

The course went reasonably well the first year and I have continued with minor tweaking for seven years so far, serving 70 teams comprising about 420 students.

To assess whether we were meeting our learning goals, we used individual tests, individual and group analyses of research papers, and a group research proposal. The tests were very challenging compared to my former tests (more open-ended questions). The questions presented data sets with the purposefully vague instructions: Draw appropriate conclusions. The students were required to describe why the experiment was done, then interpret the results accordingly. Having had ample in-class practice, most students were reasonably successful, although there was still a range of scores on each test allowing me to distinguish high performance from average or low performance. In comparison, under my former lecture method, only one or two exceptional students were able to answer similar test questions.

In addition to problems and tests, the students also did two paper analyses, one as a team and one individually. These involved reading a research article and answering a series of questions about the methods used and the interpretation of data (I assigned the papers). We did the group paper before the individual one so that weaker students would learn to recognize and produce excellent answers. Finally, the final exam was in the form of a group research proposal. During the extended final exam time, each group produced an outline of a research plan on a specific biological scenario. The plans included the question being addressed, several specific aims, a list of experiments, some hypothetical results and possible interpretation. The outlines were recorded on overhead transparencies and presented to the class.

Students were suspicious of TBL in the beginning, but they ended up enjoying the class and commenting positively on evaluations. Even at 8:30 a.m., no one fell asleep. Several students admitted that they finally learned how to study, having been forced into it by the regular RATs and graded assignments. Based on the types of test questions that were dismal failures in the past, I have seen a dramatic improvement in thinking and application skills. Finally, the final exam/research proposal confirms that most of the students have met the goals. Although this is a group assignment and is part of the group grade, for two years I experimented with having the students write individual responses first. To my delight more than half of the students made reasonable proposals on their own. With the input of team members, all of the group proposals passed muster.

One of the less quantifiable but pleasing aspects of TBL was watching students grow and mature. For example, one year the class included a seasoned high school chemistry teacher who was taking courses for biology certification. Because of her confidence, Alice was usually the first person to start the conversation, and because of her age and experience, the undergraduate students in her group automatically assumed that anything she offered was correct. Unfortunately, they failed to realize that they were actually better able to propose solutions, especially at the beginning, because their introductory biology knowledge was decades more recent than hers. When Alice's opinion was the minority one, they sweated to make her (sometimes incorrect) solution work, becoming quite frustrated when the problem refused to be solved that way. When I checked in with the group, I asked them to lay out the different options and helped them see, to their surprise, that the younger student's alternative proposal would work better. Fortunately Alice was perceptive and gracious; she backed off from being the starter, waiting patiently for another to begin the process. In the end the team was consistently doing high-quality work, including Alice, and the undergraduates gained a valuable boost in self-confidence. Overall, I have very much enjoyed watching the maturing process. I would be much less aware of the students' development if I was stuck lecturing all the time. Some bright but quiet students gained self-confidence and respect from teammates because of their high-quality work. In a lecture-based course, no one would have known the extent of their abilities. Likewise, a few well-meaning but overbearing students learned to curb their responses to avoid inadvertently sounding arrogant. In both cases, the teamwork and the peer evaluations were instrumental in the students' growth processes.

On the final course evaluations, the student comments were mostly positive and have continued to be so. For example, "The increased interaction allowed me to understand different perspectives," "The group work helped to make everything easier & more enjoyable; it was a welcome break from lectures," "I greatly enjoyed the emphasis on group work and problems, it forces you to keep up with the material. I also liked that tests were only 1/2 of the total grade. I do not test well and it really helped to have other points in my grade," "This class gave me back my confidence that I can be a science major. I wish all my science classes were built around discussion." There are still some students who prefer lecture to group interaction but they are in the clear minority.

STRUGGLES

For me, probably the most challenging issue with TBL is grading, especially considering national trends in grade inflation. What proportion of the grade comes from group work and what proportion comes from individual work? I struggle with this every year, changing the relative proportions from time to time in an effort to be fair but maintain appropriate rigor. I have not yet been courageous enough to let the students determine the grade weights as recommended by Larry Michaelsen, but I might do so in the future.

Among about 70 teams over seven years, I have had only two disappointing groups. In one group, the best student displayed passive-resistant behavior; although she was highly capable of doing the work on her own, she was completely unwilling to contribute more than body heat to the group process. In contrast, the most vocal team member was very assertive and confident, but her confidence was unfounded;

compared to her peers, her knowledge base and preparation were inadequate. Between these two extremes, the group struggled consistently to provide reasonable solutions within a decent time interval, and I believe that the remaining team members would have fared better in other groups.

I had a similar disappointing outcome last year with one group composed entirely of introverts. At times, one or two of them tried valiantly to step up to the plate, but they were consistently discouraged by negative responses from the rest of the team, even when I confirmed outright that they were headed in the right direction. Despite high grades in previous courses, repeated affirmation from me, and even a specific pep talk after class one day, they were always well behind the other groups in timing and quality. Although they made noticeable improvement from beginning to end, their effectiveness remained lower than average. I suspect that some of those students would have learned more and earned higher grades in other teams.

Recently I noticed an interesting shift in group dynamics. For five of the past seven years, the typical group interaction went something like this: When working on comprehensive questions, the teams would spend a few minutes discussing various approaches and clarifying details with me as needed. As soon as a correct approach was confirmed, all brains focused on that solution, and the problem was finished in three to five minutes. Then they would move on to the next one. This year, I noticed a dramatic decrease in the number of problems that we could solve in a day. The teams were busy talking, and they were staying on task, but less work was getting accomplished. One particular day I prodded the slowest group and helped its members decide on a correct approach. To my surprise, 10 minutes later they were still debating strategies and I had to step in to make them finish the problem. I was very concerned that their slow pace indicated unusually poor understanding of the concepts (or failure to agree for some insidious reason). After class I talked with some of the team members. It turned out that they fully comprehended the approved solution. Nevertheless, before they could apply this solution, each person who had started with a different idea had to justify why he or she had initially been wrong. In other words, the class time became a therapy session instead of a task session! After a stern reminder about the purpose of in-class work and a move from the back of the room to the front, this team actually blossomed into an effective group. The take-home lesson for me was that I needed to be very clear about how we work together in class; apparently these skills are not ordinary to the current generation of students. In response, I now spend more time in the beginning describing appropriate group dynamics and my specific expectations.

CONCLUSION

In conclusion, I have been more than satisfied with the transformation of the genetics course. The students gain a greater understanding of principles of inheritance and the application of genetic technology to real-world situations. One external measure of our overall success in the preparation of premedical students is that our average scores on the biological sciences section of the MCAT are consistently above the national average. In addition, since I write a great many letters of recommendation for students aspiring to professional schools, I am able to comment accurately about a student's ability to work well with others—something that would be hard to do from just a lecture-based course. Professional schools value an applicant's academic record, but also they look for applicants who can work with others collaboratively and respectfully.

CHAPTER 12

Team-Based Learning in an Introductory Biochemistry Class

A First-Time User's Perspective

Teresa A. Garrett

I first learned about team-based learning (TBL) in April 2006 at the American Society for Biochemistry and Molecular Biology annual meeting in San Francisco. At that meeting there was a poster session dedicated to science education and teaching methods. Because of my roles in medical school and undergraduate science education at Duke University I attended the poster session and met Scott Zimmerman from Missouri State University. He had a poster on the use of TBL for teaching a physiology class of more than 100 students (Zimmerman & Timson, 2006). As he explained the method and the results I was intrigued. I ordered *Team-Based Learning: A Transformative Use of Small Groups in College Teaching* (Michaelsen, Knight, & Fink, 2004) and began thinking about how to integrate TBL into my teaching.

In this chapter I present my initial experiences with TBL. I tried TBL in my class without ever attending a TBL conference or observing another teacher using TBL. I had the conversation with Scott Zimmerman, the TBL book, a Web site (http://www.ou.edu/idp/teamlearning/), and a colleague at Duke who had experience with TBL as my resources. So far, I have used TBL in an undergraduate science class and have begun to use it in a medical school course. Here I share my initial experiences, both good and bad, with the hope that they will encourage others who have never used TBL, to dive in and just give it a try.

WHY I WANTED TO TRY TBL

I was interested in TBL for several reasons. The pedagogical reasons outlined in *Team-Based Learning: A Transformative Use of Small Groups in College Teaching* and elsewhere in this volume certainly apply. In particular, I was drawn to the way the TBL teaching strategy combined learning the course content with team building and directly using the course content to solve problems. In addition, I wanted to de-emphasize memorization, emphasize critical thinking, and engage the students in a fun, active learning experience.

I was frustrated about the enormous amount of rote memorization the students in my Introduction to Biochemistry class seemed to be doing. Science students must spend a certain amount of time learning the vocabulary and paradigms that pervade biochemistry. However, with easy access to vast stores of information via the Internet and other sources I felt that I must reconsider whether rote memorization of biochemical pathways is necessary or even useful for understanding the core concepts I wanted my students to understand. Many of the biochemical pathways of the cell are much easier to learn if one thinks through them, applying previously mastered knowledge of chemistry and organic chemistry.

In conjunction with de-emphasizing memorization, I wanted to emphasize applied, critical thinking. With the vast amounts of information that are readily available, the need to develop critical thinking skills becomes even more important. Students need to be able to critically evaluate the available information and apply it to problems in new and interesting ways. Also, this science class does not have a hands-on laboratory component. I felt that TBL could become a mechanism by which I could have the students critically analyze actual laboratory data without a formal lab class.

I was also interested in using TBL because it seemed fun. I love engaging students in science, helping them get excited about the material, and interested in learning more about the subject. This can be hard to do when you stand at the board and lecture class after class. I saw TBL as a way to break up the monotony and liven up the classroom a bit.

GETTING STARTED USING TBL

My undergraduate course, Introduction to Biochemistry, runs in a six-week summer session. The class meets for 75 minutes every day and covers protein structure and function, basic enzyme kinetics, metabolism, and nucleic acid biochemistry. In the past I have taught the course entirely lecturing at the blackboard. A similar course, with significantly larger enrollment, is taught by departmental faculty in the fall semester using a similar format and following a similar syllabus. No one in the department had ever tried TBL, though it had been introduced in the medical school for a period of time before I began teaching at Duke. Several colleagues questioned whether the same amount of content could be covered in the same time frame. Others wondered why I wanted to change from lecturing, a teaching method that was working for me. Nonetheless I was intrigued to see if I could improve my teaching using TBL, and so I pushed forward.

For this first time using TBL, I planned five TBL sessions distributed throughout the six weeks of the course. After introducing the TBL concept to the class on the first day, I separated the class into teams. I chose to divide the 50-student class into five groups of seven and two groups of eight. To divide the students into teams, I had them line up around the perimeter of the room according to major; first biology majors then chemistry, engineering, math, and so on. The only manipulation I did to this initial lineup was to pull students who had already obtained a bachelor's degree to the end of the line. The students then counted off and gathered into their teams to provide a roster for their team, get to know each other, and take a team photo.

I considered other ways to divide the students into teams including randomly assigning teams or giving a pretest and using the pretest score to make the teams. In the end I chose a method that was completely transparent to the students. I felt it was important for the students to see that I tried to make each team equivalent. Once the teams were formed I did not alter the teams to balance for gender or ethnicity. This resulted in one team that had six males and one female. After consulting with the young woman to make sure that she was comfortable with the team composition, I left the teams as they were.

In general, I followed the standard TBL format for each session. Before each TBL session, the students were given a reading assignment from the textbook. It usually was between 15 and 35 pages from *Lehninger Principles of Biochemistry* (Nelson & Cox, 2005). At the start of each session the students were asked to sit with their teams, and each team was given a team folder. I taped team pictures onto the front of each folder to facilitate handing them out. Each folder contained the individual Readiness Assurance Tests (IRATS), individual answer sheets, a group answer sheet, group application questions, and a set of response letters for simultaneous reporting of the answers to the group Readiness Assurance Tests (GRATs) and group application exercise questions. In addition, I used the folder to hand back homework or exams to team members.

The TBL sessions began with an IRAT of six to eight multiple-choice questions over the assigned reading. I did not make these questions exceedingly difficult. I told the students that if they had carefully read the chapter they would have no problem on the IRAT. I wanted them to prepare for the TBL sessions without becoming overly stressed out about a short quiz. In essence I wanted the TBL to be a positive experience for the students. These assessments were open book but time limited, such that a student who did not prepare would not be able to look up the answers in the time allowed. After collecting the answer sheets, the students did the GRAT, the same test as the IRAT. We reviewed the answers as a class using the response letters, cleared up any ambiguities about the assessment, and moved to the group application.

Almost all the group application exercises had a component of experimental data analysis. In some exercises, I used data from the literature or from the laboratory where I work. In other cases, I made up data to fit the application problem more closely than what I could find in the literature. Using fabricated data allowed me to carefully control what the students were analyzing, keeping them focused on the specific concepts and questions that I wanted to emphasize and preventing confusion that could arise from analyzing real experimental data.

During the group application exercise I went around to the teams to answer questions, give clarification, and challenge their thinking. It was during this component that I could really see that the students were thinking and applying their knowledge.

This is the part of TBL that is most gratifying to me as a teacher. The room is buzzing with discussion, hand waving, peering at data, and flipping through the book to come to the correct answer. After seeing this there is no doubt that this is *active* learning.

The first TBL session on the second day of class I had to deal with a problem common to many people trying to use TBL: the classroom setup. I teach in a fixed-seating lecture hall that accommodates about 125 students. I encouraged the students to sit in such a way that they were all able to participate in the team discussions. One team ended up sitting in two rows with two people in the front and five in the back so that three people at the end were just sitting there, facing forward looking annoyed and not participating in the discussion. It was not that the other team members were actively excluding them from the discussion; it was that the physical orientation of the people hindered their participation. I approached the team and had them all stand up and reorient themselves so they could all participate in the discussion. From then on that team functioned quite well together.

While most of the group application exercises had multiple-choice answers, I usually made the last one or two questions of the exercise short-answer questions. After going over the multiple-choice questions in class using the response letters, the teams shared the different answers they had for the short-answer questions. Following the class I graded the group application exercise, including the short-answer questions, scanned the team answer sheets, and posted the file to the electronic course blackboard. In this way everyone in the class benefited from the other teams answers and any comments I had. I included these more opened questions to try to gauge the depth of thinking that was going on in the group discussions. Others who have used problem-based learning in advanced biochemistry courses have used opened-ended problems in which the final answers were posted on poster board around the room for the other groups to grade and evaluate (White, 2002). This first time around I was not able to see how to incorporate that technique into the TBL sessions and may use that technique in the future.

RESULTS OF USING TBL

I did not collect data charting performance on standardized exams or even enough data to say that student grades were higher when taught using TBL versus lectures, given that I have only been teaching this class for three years total (two years entirely lecture, one year TBL enhanced). I do have my personal impression of how it went, course reviews, and the results of a single survey question given at the end of class.

My overall impression of this first try at TBL was very positive. I looked forward to the TBL sessions as a break from lecturing. I was energized by the students' participation in the TBL process. It was fun and exciting and challenging. I enjoyed getting more thought-provoking questions from my students and seeing them discuss ideas with each other during class. It was also fun to watch my students actively seeking answers to problems rather than passively observing a lecture. I will definitely use TBL in the future.

As the instructor, my overall course evaluations were improved from previous years. My score for "quality of instruction" went up from 4.16 to 4.69 points out of 5 possible. Given that this was the third year of my teaching this course I can't say for certain that the increase was because of my implementation of TBL in the course or simply the product of more experience. I know that I found the course more enjoyable to teach.

The overall class average compared to previous years was three percentage points higher when I used TBL. Because this was my first experience using TBL I did not make the IRATs exceedingly difficult. The students generally scored well on the group application exercises. With the TBL portion of the grade at 12.5% this could be inflating this year's grades slightly. However, when I compare exam scores between the two years, the average score on the exams was also about three percentage points higher. It will take more time for me to really tell if student performance is enhanced in a statistically significant way.

In addition to the university evaluation, I generally ask a few extra questions that are specific for the particular class. In this year's supplemental survey I asked about TBL. Figure 12.1 shows the responses to the statement "I felt the Team-Based Learning activities enhanced my learning activities." Most of the comments that the students added were positive. Some comments reflected the increased critical thinking that was taking place in the classroom. For example, one student commented, "The Team-based learning forced me to think outside the box and encouraged independent learning." Others touched on the team-building process, commenting, "Being in a group with several different majors made each approach to every TBL diverse. Everyone brought something different to the group." Most of the criticism surrounded not knowing what material from the TBL session would be on the exam. "TBL was enjoyable but when it came to review for exams it was hard to know which details to focus on from those sections," was one student's comment. Thanks to these constructive comments I will be able to improve the use of TBL in the future.

LESSONS LEARNED

In my first try with TBL I encountered a few problems that I will address in future classes. Some of the problems and possible solutions are presented below.

PROBLEM #1: Fixed-seat lecture hall hindering team development. As related above, teaching in a fixed-seat amphitheater makes it more difficult for the students to interact effectively.

SOLUTION: I will continue to be on the lookout for two things: a classroom more amenable to the TBL process, and for teams that are not functioning properly because of the physical constraints of the classroom.

FIGURE 12.1
Student Response to the Statement: I Felt the Team-Based Learning Activities Enhanced My Learning Activities

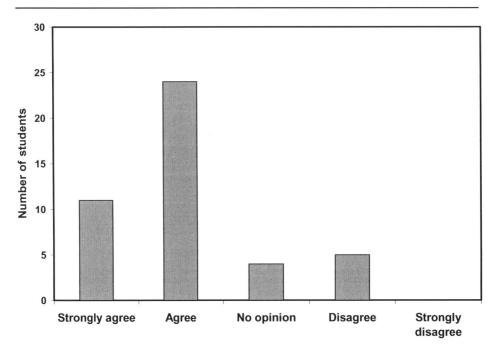

PROBLEM #2: Students weren't sure what material in the assigned reading would be covered during the TBL session. As mentioned above this was a recurring criticism during the class and on the course evaluations.

SOLUTION: Make a TBL prep study guide that outlines the core concepts and goals of the session. This should help focus the students' efforts on the material that is the most relevant.

PROBLEM #3: Students weren't sure what material from the TBL prep and the TBL session would be emphasized on the exams. Again, this was a recurring criticism.

SOLUTION: Supplement in-class reviews with a handout of notes emphasizing the core material.

PROBLEM #4: The TBL session didn't cover all of the material that the students were expected to know. Often when preparing for a TBL session, I had what I considered to be a particularly interesting problem for the group application exercise. More than once I made the mistake of focusing the group application on this problem so much that the other core concepts weren't addressed in the TBL session. For example, the molecular basis of phenylketonuria is an excellent problem involving amino acid catabolism. However, focusing on the problems associated with the degradation of a single amino acid didn't cover important biochemical concepts of nitrogen metabolism, such as the urea cycle.

SOLUTION: Prepare group application exercise questions with the goals of the session clearly in mind. Based on discussions with Larry Michaelson and Dean Parmelee, I will try to draw in associated concepts through carefully designed questions in which discussion or understanding of those other concepts must take place to effectively answer the question. For the example above, I will design questions with multiple-choice options that make the students think about the urea cycle and where it could affect phenylalanine metabolism even though the application exercise focuses on phenylketonuria.

PROBLEM #5: Not finishing the session in 75 minutes. Because of the syllabus that I was following and the need to work within the allotted class time, I need to make sure that the TBL sessions fit from start to finish in a single class session of 75 minutes.

SOLUTIONS: There are a few straightforward solutions to this problem. First, reduce the number of questions in the group application exercise. As I had to learn how many questions constitute a one-hour exam, I must also learn how many questions constitute a group application exercise for a 75-minute TBL session. Second, implement some tricks I learned during a visit to Wright State University's Boonshoft School of Medicine. In their TBL sessions, they project a timer using a document camera. The students know how much time is allotted for each part of the TBL session and work accordingly. In addition, each team had flagpoles and the students post flags atop their flagpole to signal that they were done with an activity. If the entire class finished before the allotted time the class moved on to the next section of the TBL. These are great ideas for keeping the session on time and moving along and I will implement them the next time I teach a class using TBL.

In the future I will also experiment with slightly smaller groups, perhaps no more than six students per group. With 50 students I would have six groups of six and two groups of seven. Some students felt the groups were too large, so I will try keeping them at five to seven students. I will try using the Immediate Feedback-Assessment Technique (IF-AT) answer sheets for the GRAT. If the team doesn't come up with the correct answer it has a chance to regroup and discuss where the teammates went wrong and try again for reduced credit. I would also like to institute peer review at the end of the class. The students will evaluate their team members on coming to class prepared and participation in the team's work. Their TBL grade would be scaled by a factor related to this peer review score.

IMPLEMENTING TBL IN BASIC SCIENCE EDUCATION AT THE MEDICAL SCHOOL

In addition to teaching undergraduates in the summer session, I am the course coordinator for the first class of the Duke Medical School curriculum, Molecules and

Cells. This is a fully integrated six-week course that covers basic science concepts of biochemistry, genetics, and cell biology. It consists of more than 110 student contact hours with more than 40 faculty members contributing to lectures, disease and patient-centered clinical correlations, histology labs, and review sessions. My role has been to coordinate the course by attending all lectures, facilitating review sessions, and assembling exams. Having sat through the course three years in a row, I thought TBL would be a good addition to this course because it would reinforce critical thinking skills and add more active learning to the course.

The Molecules and Cells course directors supported implementing some TBL into the course as a way to supplement and integrate various concepts and basic science paradigms. For example, a TBL on Huntington's disease integrated concepts of DNA replication, protein structure, protein folding, and human genetics while having the students critically analyze clinical and basic science data.

We divided the class up similarly to the undergraduate biochemistry course, according to undergraduate major. I made two modifications for this postbaccalaureate group of students; anyone who had a postgraduate degree was moved to the end of the line regardless of major, and a subset of pathology assistants program students (six students total, who take this class as part of their curriculum) were kept together as a team.

Because of the lessons I learned with the undergraduate class earlier in the year, I was careful to have the goals and objectives of each TBL session clearly laid out for the class. Before each TBL session the students were given guidelines for their preparations that included attending class and/or watching the streaming video of the class and perhaps a short reading from a textbook. This seemed to help alleviate problems #2 and #3 above.

This class was more than twice the size of the undergraduate course; there are 105 students. For each TBL session I partnered with an additional instructor, well versed in the TBL session content. This meant there were two faculty members to answer questions during the group application exercise. This worked out very well for this size class. The number of questions that the students had kept both of us very busy for nearly the entire duration of the group application exercise.

We had similar challenges because of the physical restraints of the amphitheater used by the class. The amphitheater was fixed seating and really not large enough to give the 15 teams enough room to spread out. In addition, the room got very loud once everyone was discussing the GRAT and group application exercise. Several students who learned and worked better in quieter conditions complained about the distracting level of noise. I am not sure how to solve these problems in the future. The fixed-seating issues can be worked around with careful monitoring of the teams to make sure that the seating is not hindering team development. The size of the amphitheater and the noise level are more difficult problems to solve. We could divide the class into two TBL sessions with about 50 students each. Two successive TBL sessions may be taxing to the instructors and hard to schedule in the very compact schedule of the course.

Because the IRAT and group application exercise questions were being written and used for the first time, the students found some ambiguity in the wording of some questions very frustrating. This, of course, is par for the course when you are using new multiple-choice questions. The students have a tendency to read into the questions in ways that I, personally, cannot predict. Each year as the questions are revised and fine-tuned in response to student criticism this should be less and less of a problem.

These first steps into using TBL in the Medical School Molecules and Cells course have been positive. From course reviews, many students felt that TBL enhanced their learning and had suggestions for where it could be improved. The instructors that I worked with appreciated the change of pace from lectures and the increased interaction with the students. I plan to improve and expand upon the use of TBL in this class in the future by gradually adding new sessions to the curriculum as students and faculty become more accustomed to the TBL process.

FINAL THOUGHTS

My initial experiences with TBL have been amazing. Through this process I was able to actually see that the students were engaged in critical thinking and teamwork. As a teacher who loves to see students get excited about science, this was a very fulfilling experience. Their enthusiasm for learning permeated the room during the group application exercise discussion periods. They asked interesting, thoughtful, discerning questions and had insights into the material that I would have never known about except through the TBL process.

I hope that my experiences will encourage others to jump in and try TBL in their teaching. You don't need to attend a workshop or have been a student in a TBL session (though I am sure that it wouldn't hurt) before you can give it a try. The TBL book and Web site are great resources for getting started using TBL. If you can, contact someone who is using TBL to discuss the logistics and help troubleshoot any issues that are holding you back.

Finally, I would like to acknowledge my students. They were open to trying this new teaching strategy. I encouraged them to give me comments and criticisms, and they did so with the utmost professionalism. My teaching and use of TBL will continue to improve because of their openness and enthusiasm for learning. I am proud to have partnered with them on this adventure into TBL.

REFERENCES

Michaelsen, L. K., Knight, A. B., & Fink, L. D. (2004). *Team-based learning: A transformative use of small groups in college teaching*. Sterling, VA: Stylus Publishing.

Nelson, D. L., & Cox, M. M. (2005). *Lehninger principles of biochemistry* (4th ed.). New York: W. H. Freeman.

White, H. B. (2002). Plants versus animals in the dining hall: A problem-based learning problem. *Biochemistry and Molecular Biology Education, 30*(5), 315–221.

Zimmerman, S. D., & Timson, B. F. (2006). Team-based learning improves performance in a physiology laboratory course. *The Federation of American Societies for Experimental Biology Journal, 20*, A17.

CHAPTER 13

Using Team-Based Learning as a Substitute for Lectures in a Required Undergraduate Nursing Course

Michele C. Clark

My first exposure to team-based learning (TBL) was in 2004. I was discussing with a colleague my concern about the overall drop in our nursing graduates' National Council Licensure Examination (NCLEX) scores. My colleague, a physician, had been piloting and evaluating a new teaching modality, TBL, which was supported by a grant from the Fund for the Improvement of Postsecondary Education (FIPSE). She informed me that for 18 months, the FIPSE grant project supported 40 courses, ranging from preclinical to clinical medical education, one residency program, and three clinical courses in the physician assistant's program. She reported that in classes where she used the pilot TBL model, her students' academic performance was equal to or better than the performance of others in classes using lecture-based content delivery.

At the time, I was creating a new required course combining nursing theory and clinical elements; this course grouped contents of two other classes that were focused on the older adult and on case management for vulnerable populations. The content had been organized around nine modules that would be supported by nine formal lectures. My enthusiasm in creating these lectures was dampened by my disappointment that many students were not consistently attending the lectures. Meanwhile, those students who did attend were not reading the required background texts, making it difficult for them to engage in the class or to ask meaningful questions during the lecture. As the semester progressed in this traditional lecture format class, students were often unprepared to participate in any class discussion. Furthermore, there didn't seem to be a relationship between the students' final grade and class attendance.

These reasons propelled me to ask my colleague, who was using TBL, to present a workshop on this new teaching strategy. The faculty participated actively in this engaging workshop. Despite their enthusiasm during the workshop, the nursing faculty were skeptical that a technique that required students to master basic content before class was realistic; in fact, many thought that this experiment was doomed to failure. More troublesome to the faculty was the amount of content that each student team would need to cover during each lecture. They questioned the students' ability to pick out the material needed for basic safety in nursing practice. As an educator, I found this to be a problematic assumption. If students were unable to read material and pick out the areas that were most pertinent for practice, then how were they going to continue to improve their practice with relevant readings?

These questions and concerns led the faculty to evaluate student readings, including the number of pages students were assigned in each course. When faculty realized that students' weekly assignments of one or two chapters often added up to 50 to 60 pages, totaling 600–800 pages per course by the end of the semester, they began to understand why students were not reading. Such assignments were impossible to complete. This important discussion led to a more focused reading assignment. Faculty decided what was most pertinent for the students' success with the content. Appropriate, more streamlined reading assignments are critical for the success of this teaching strategy.

After some discussion of the potential benefits and problems with this teaching modality, the nursing faculty decided to use TBL to teach four modules within the new eight-module course called Case Management for Older Adults. This required course ran seven weeks, with approximately 70 third-semester junior nursing students registered.

To introduce the students to TBL, students participated in a TBL experience during their orientation to the course. We presented a short lecture explaining the theory and components of TBL and informed the students that there would be a short quiz on the content following the lecture. After the lecture, we formed 10 teams made up of seven students; the teams were to remain intact throughout the seven weeks. To ensure that students' resources (work experience, intelligence, class preparation time) were equally distributed among the groups, groups were divided using predetermined criteria related to work schedules, parenting responsibilities, and course load. These criteria were chosen based on our previous experiences with students and our feeling that these unique life experiences would produce diverse groups.

We decided not to use academic performance data because we wanted the students to be aware of how the groups were formed. We felt that disclosure of our method prevented students from thinking that there was an ulterior motive in forming the groups. Also everyone had an equal and fair chance of being placed in a group. Despite the fact that we didn't consider grades in forming our groups, each group had a good variation in race, gender, and academic ability. We chose not to give the groups time to get acquainted because it was our belief that the students had been in the nursing program for two semesters and should be familiar with each other.

After the groups were formed, students were given a 10-item individual Readiness Assurance Test (IRAT) on the content presented in class. Students were given about 15 minutes to complete the quiz and were asked to pass them in. They were then asked to go into their preformed groups to take the quiz again, but this time with the assistance of their group members. We then seated all the groups together and asked the groups to work within their teams on the group Readiness Assurance Tests (GRATs). We handed out one Immediate Feedback-Assessment Technique (IF-AT) scoring sheet to each group and instructed the students to scratch off their choices for the multiple-choice quiz.

Students often complain about group work so we were surprised at the active participation of each of the groups during the GRAT exercise. The noise level in the classroom was high, as everyone was participating in deciding on the best answer for each item in the GRAT. When we walked around the class to see what the groups were discussing, we found them freely disagreeing with each other and actively explaining their thoughts. We were a little surprised at the activity in the class and were not sure if this enthusiastic engagement would be maintained when the course content was being presented during the next week and the IRAT and GRAT were graded.

The final component of TBL introduced during this orientation time was the application exercise. During this exercise students are given a scenario based on the content they have learned and then given three to four multiple-choice questions to decide on how to answer as a group. The questions require more critical thinking skills and often ask for the best answer rather than the right answer.

The content for the application exercise, how to break bad news, was familiar content to nursing students, and the students were active and vocal in supporting their choice of one of the four possible answers for each question. However, there was much more engagement during the GRATs than the application exercise. We felt this may have been because the format of the application exercise requires student groups to defend their answers to the whole class. However, we were interested in seeing if students became more comfortable with this skill as they participated in this exercise throughout the semester.

At the end of orientation, we informed the class that four of eight course modules would use TBL and that they needed to review their syllabus for the TBL times, as students would be expected to come to the class prepared. We also asked them to review in the syllabus how this experience would be graded; we would discuss the grading in the next class. We finished this orientation by asking the students if they had any questions or concerns about this new teaching-learning strategy. The class voiced some excitement about this type of learning and there were no questions. Some of the students' comments were, "This was fun," and "Class went by so quickly today."

OUR FIRST EXPERIENCE WITH TBL

The nursing course Case Management of the Older Adult and Other Vulnerable Populations included an individual and group RAT for four of the eight modules. Since one of the goals for employing this new teaching strategy was to improve critical thinking skills, application exercises related to the content of the course were also used for the four modules.

EXPLAINING THE GRADING SYSTEM

During the second class for the course, faculty explained the grading system that would be applied to the modules using TBL. Students were informed that a total of 12% of their grade would be calculated from their scores on their IRAT and GRAT. The scores would be divided up so that their IRAT would be 1% of their grade, while their GRAT would be 3% of their total grade. We decided to give more weight to the GRAT because we wanted to build group cohesion and we felt that if the group grade was worth more than the individual grade, group members would be more motivated to work as a group and hold each individual member accountable for preparing for class.

IRATs AND GRATs

When students were aware that there were consequences to their performance on the IRATs and GRATs, they voiced some concern about not knowing how to organize their reading to prepare for these tests. We assured them that the reading had been considerably shortened and that they might try outlining their readings to help structure their studying. Despite the students' initial concerns, our first class went well and the students were pretty active in class. The students initially took a 15-item IRAT that focused on the content of the assigned readings. Each student was given a Scantron form; they wrote their name and student ID on it. The class was given 20 minutes to complete the IRAT. They turned in their Scantron forms and proceeded to their groups to complete their GRAT. While students were involved in completing their GRAT, faculty graded the students' IRAT. We have found that grading the IRAT is very beneficial in evaluating what content the students are unclear about.

In our first classes, we waited until everyone had completed their GRAT before we progressed to a short lecture or the application exercise. Some students complained that because some groups were slow to complete their GRAT, other groups had empty time that was wasted with the waiting. For this reason, we limited the time to complete the GRAT to 40 minutes. This worked well, and students later stated that they felt that the time in the class was put to better use toward learning complex material.

When the GRAT was completed, we asked each group to report its scores. We put each group GRAT score on the board so that each group could evaluate how it was doing in relation to the other groups. This simple act facilitated individual accountability. In fact when this activity was skipped in error, one group member stood up independently and placed his group score on the board.

APPEALS

Past experience with students arguing about questions made us hesitant to include the grade appeal process in the TBL pilot experience, in particular appealing a question or questions on the GRAT; however, in the end, we did set up clear grade appeal criteria similar to those suggested by Michaelsen and his colleagues (Michaelsen, Knight, & Fink, 2004).

We informed our students they could appeal a particular question if they could identify that it was factually wrong based on their text, or they could appeal the question if it was confusing because of wording. This was the only time students were allowed to use their references or text. Thus, we required students to provide the citation documenting their answer as correct, or to rewrite the question to make it clearer. There was no classroom discussion of the appeals. Students completed the appeals sheet addressing one or both of the criteria and passed it in at the end of class. We informed the groups that even if a question was incorrectly scored, only the groups who appealed a question would actually get credit for it.

At the beginning of the class, all the groups appealed questions, usually in an argumentative fashion, and citations were often unrelated to the questions. As the lead faculty member, I did review all appeals and gave the student written feedback regarding whether his or her arguments warranted credit for the selected question. After my initial feedback, students were more discriminating on appealing questions; appeals became more thoughtful and were usually supported with citations from the readings or text. Despite our initial trepidation, this appeals process became a powerful learning experience for the students as well as the faculty.

SHORT, FOCUSED LECTURE

When we started using TBL after reporting the scores for the GRAT, we would go immediately to the application exercise—an exercise where students would apply the content they learned to a case study or clinical situation. We soon realized that after students completed their GRAT, and we had finished grading the IRAT, we had an opportunity to clear up any confusion students had on the content. We often saw a pattern of missed items on the IRAT and used this as a guide to either lecture or use Socratic questioning to clear up any confusion on the content.

APPLICATION EXERCISES

Recent trends in nursing education demand that exit goals for graduating seniors include critical thinking skills and problem-solving skills for complex health care situations (Garrett, Schoener, & Hood, 1996). We were dismayed that most of our students were depending on the PowerPoint handouts as the primary learning material for the course, and we felt that this might have been one of the many reasons that our NCLEX scores were going down. We hoped that the application exercises in TBL could help us to prepare students to learn problem-solving strategies to address complex nursing care situations that are frequently being presented on graduate nurse licensure exams in the form of case scenarios.

We understood from our readings on TBL that our application exercises needed to allow our students to use the content they had acquired with higher-level cognitive skills. Therefore, we decided that all application exercises would be based on case studies representing complicated clinical situations. Scenarios needed to include enough information to allow students to make a decision but be complex enough to generate discussion from the group. We also decided not to grade the application exercises.

We felt that we faced some challenges in building group cohesion and maintaining accountability. To address these issues, we followed the three procedures coined by Michaelsen as the three *S*s (Michaelsen et al., 2004): same problem, specific choice, and simultaneous reporting.

We found the three *S*s to be essential in stimulating thoughtful discussion both within groups and between groups. Each of the 10 groups received the same case study, including a number of questions in which the groups had to choose a specific answer (choice). We developed our questions so that all the responses had some possible fit, but when all the presented information was taken into consideration, one answer was better than the other choices.

In order to allow for simultaneous reporting, we presented each group with a set of cards printed with an A, B, C, D, or E. When students were in their groups, they were required to pick one answer to the questions, which were numbered from A to E. Initially some groups complained that they had two answers because the group couldn't decide on an answer. At those times, we stopped the class, giving the group three minutes to make a choice. Then we would call the groups' attention back to the class. We would then read the scenarios, starting with the first question. We would ask the class at the count of three to raise their cards printed with the letter that represented their answer.

Once all options were read for one question, we often had a lively discussion between groups. Faculty also gained insight about how students analyzed the scenarios as well as the problem-solving skills they used to decide on the best answer for the question. However, when all groups picked the same answer to the application question, we were still able to generate a class discussion by asking a particular group why it thought its option was better than, for example, option B. A second group might be asked why it thought its option was superior to option C. This allowed the faculty and students to evaluate how groups came to their clinical decisions. Initially students complained that they felt the instructors were too challenging when they were questioned during the application exercises. This was discovered during midterm evaluations when faculty asked for the strengths and challenges of this new teaching modality. Therefore, faculty became mindful of reinforcing students' answers and highlighting for the class the problem-solving strategies that were appropriate even if the group's choice of options was not the best answer. Conversely, when students demonstrated a lack of understanding of the content or poor problem-solving strategies, faculty encouraged other groups who chose better options to explain how they used the content to come to their conclusions.

Students felt the application exercises were the most helpful in their learning experience but often reported frustration because coming to the conclusion of the best answer often took time and informed discussion with all members of the group. Students expressed fears they would not be able to answer these types of questions in their exams. Faculty had to reassure the students that these exercises were to facilitate students' learning. In contrast, the purpose of the exam questions was to evaluate students' knowledge of content and problem-solving skills. (See Appendix 13.A.)

LESSONS LEARNED WHEN USING TBL

Preparing for a TBL class takes a significant amount of preparation. RATs and application exercises require thought and a significant investment of time. Since the readings are where the students get the information to prepare them for the TBL experience, readings must be assigned so that students can focus on the areas that are most important to learn. For us, this required decreasing the reading assignments and evaluating which readings would give the students the information they needed to know to be successful. We were unaware of the time commitment in preparing to use TBL. Initially using TBL for half of the course content gave us time in developing the structure, learning exercises, and tools necessary to be successful. As well, students must be helped on how to move through the text and organize the material for study. Students were not reading and were unsure of how to approach the material without a lecture or PowerPoint to guide them. We spent time in many classes talking about the readings and how to organize them to study for the following class.

Students expressed concern that they would not be able to get the adequate information from the readings but felt they also needed lectures to supplement their learning. We were unable to convince a segment of the class that it was getting adequate information to be successful in the class. However, when the class grades on the midterm and final exam demonstrated the same type of grade spread that was similar with other undergraduate students taking the same course, most students felt confident that their learning was comparable to learning in previous classes.

Having the students experience TBL during their course orientation was extremely helpful. Since students were not graded during this experience, it was rather informal and fun but did not deviate from the structure necessary for TBL. Groups were formed and students learned how class would be structured with TBL. This saved considerable time and discussion. During the first class meeting, students were able to participate fully with all the components of TBL.

We were constantly trying to develop GRATs and application exercises that promoted learning and team development (Michaelsen & Richards, 2005). Though the GRAT's primary purpose is to test content, we adopted an approach that we felt was helpful. We ensured that the questions in the GRAT ranged from easy to difficult. Easy questions gave groups confidence to move through the exercise, but the more difficult questions promoted discussion that facilitated building group cohesion.

Our faculty enjoyed TBL because they felt they got to know the students better and were clearer on how they used class content to solve clinical problems. However, our student course evaluations suggested a mixed response to the TBL method: 33% liked it very much, 47% were neutral, and 20% did not like it. Nevertheless, students who used TBL reported more in-class participation than in their lecture courses (Clark, Nguyen, Bray, & Levine, in press).

We felt the mixed evaluations may have been because this course was the first to use TBL as a primary teaching strategy. Additionally, students were new to being responsible for deciding how to organize required reading so that content was learned. Most students reported depending on the lecture for organizing their learning, and that frequently readings were not completed. This is certainly troublesome when one important goal of all education programs is to develop lifelong learners. Students, however, did report that they actively prepared for their TBL classes more than for their lecture classes because of their desire to do well on the RATs.

We felt that making the learning exercises (IRAT, GRAT) worth a part of the students' final grade facilitated their commitment to not only come to class but to come prepared. We chose to give more credit to the group exercise because we felt that this would build group cohesion and provide encouragement, since the GRAT scores were always better than the IRAT scores.

CONCLUSION

We felt that the benefits of TBL far outweighed the traditional lecture format. Students in TBL were more engaged in the learning process and used more communication skills to express their arguments for an answer. This increase in communication abilities was evident to the researchers in the amount and distribution of dialogue with the instructors and with other students throughout the course. As well, TBL was useful as an instructional method for clinical content for solving complex clinical problems. More importantly, students using TBL met course objectives with fewer lectures. Though students' enthusiasm didn't match the faculty's, students did agree that they learned how to solve complex clinical problems as well as to manage the diverse experiences and personalities of group members.

Our experience with TBL demonstrates that it is a promising teaching strategy to enhance student nurse learning, and as we see the changes in our health care system that demand more and better communication within and between teams, TBL is an excellent fit.

REFERENCES

Clark, M. C., Nguyen, H. T., Bray, C., & Levine, R. (in press). Team learning in an undergraduate nursing course. *Journal of Nursing Education*.

Garret, M. L., Schoener, L., & Hood, L. (1996). Debate: A teaching strategy to improve verbal communication and critical-thinking skills. *Nurse Educator, 21*, 37–40.

Michaelsen, L. K., Knight, A. B., & Fink, L. D. (2004). *Team-based learning: A transformative use of small groups in college teaching*. Sterling, VA: Stylus Publishing.

Michaelsen, L., & Richards, B. (2005). Drawing conclusions for the "Team-Learning" literature in health-sciences education: A commentary. *Teaching and Learning in Medicine, 17*(1), 85–88.

APPENDIX 13.A

Sample Group Application Exercise: Environmental Assessment

Case: Mrs. A is a 75-year-old single woman. She retired from teaching grammar school 10 years ago and lives alone in a small cottage. She was hospitalized four weeks ago after she experienced a stroke that left her with significant left-sided weakness. After a short inpatient rehabilitation stay, she has improved in function, mobility, and strength. Nevertheless, she still has significant physical disabilities. She is able to get out of bed without assistance; with a quad cane she is a household ambulator but needs wheelchair assistance in the community. Though she is right-handed, she has minimal strength and function of her right hand and moderate strength and function in her right leg. She lives alone and is soon to be discharged. Please review the pictures of her cottage and answer the following questions.

1. All of the following are present in your home assessment. Which of the following would be your *first* priority?
   a. Use of kerosene heaters
   b. Smoking in bed
   c. Dangerous electrical wiring
   d. No smoke alarms
2. Based on the information provided in the scenario, and the pictures of the cottage you reviewed, what would be your recommendation about discharge?
   a. An assisted living center for four weeks to build up Mrs. Randall's strength.
   b. Mr. and Mrs. Randall will be fine with someone checking on them daily.
   c. Home health care to provide needed services.
   d. Remain in the hospital for another four weeks for strengthening exercises.
3. When evaluating the exterior of Mrs. Randall's home what poses the greatest threat to her safety?
   a. Width of ramp
   b. Barred windows
   c. House numbers
   d. No slide protection on the ramp
4. After assessing Mrs. Randall's dining room what would be your *first* recommendation to protect her from falls?
   a. Remove clutter on chair and floor
   b. Change rolling chairs to ones that do not move
   c. Remove throw rugs
   d. Rearrange the chairs
5. There are a variety of hazards in Mrs. Randall's bedroom. Which *one* would you want to be sure *was corrected* before you completed your home visit?
   a. Tangle of electrical cords
   b. Change position of phone
   c. Organize medications
   d. Remove the general clutter in the room

6. To assist Mrs. Randall in improving her ability to transfer safely, what would be your *first* action?
   a. Encourage recreational activities to complement rehabilitation therapies.
   b. Place a bilateral transfer enabler on her bed.
   c. Adjust the bed height specific to the resident's lower leg length.
   d. Install an accessible call bell.
7. Mrs. Randall shares with you during your home visit that she has a fear of falling. What is your major concern with this comment?
   a. Functional decline
   b. Increased morbidity
   c. Poor nutrition
   d. Social isolation

CHAPTER 14

Team-Based Learning in a Physician Assistant Program

Bob Philpot

I have taught in physician's assistant programs for many years. Early in my teaching career, I began to feel that lecturing had limitations: unless students expected a "pop quiz," they would rarely come to class having read the assignment for the day. Most students would take notes during the lecture, but I never had an idea about what they found worthy of writing down or, for that matter, what they were really learning. I devoted considerable time and effort over the years to becoming a more effective lecturer. I felt like I had improved. But I sometimes wondered if I was simply becoming more entertaining, or just getting better at keeping the students awake.

Becoming an excellent teacher is what we "academics" aspire to achieve in our careers. Designing, writing, and delivering a lecture that captures the attention and curiosity of our students can inspire them to go home and learn more. This is something we want. Discovering innovative ways to engage a class, whether with the traditional lecture or with a small-group interactive format enables us to feel that we are improving the learning opportunities for our students.

We encourage them to prepare for class. But if a student doesn't grasp a key concept, he or she may be confused for the better part of a class period. The resulting feelings of fear and helplessness can prevent learning. Team-based learning (TBL) provides them with the opportunity to clarify key concepts through interaction with their peers. Critical thinking and problem solving through teamwork facilitates this process. Students, especially those in the health professions, need us to continue to challenge them in ways that make them more thoughtful and skillful clinicians *and* clinicians who can work collaboratively with others in a variety of settings.

My first exposure to TBL was at a workshop provided as part of a faculty development program in medical education. A short introduction to TBL was followed by a reading assignment, Readiness Assurance Tests (RATs), and a group application activity. As the workshop evolved, I was intrigued by the way the structure of the strategy facilitated interaction by all of us "students." We all felt that joy of learning. Immediately, I imagined numerous ways that TBL could be integrated into the existing courses taught at our physician's assistant program.

I have now used the TBL strategy throughout an entire course as the primary mode of instruction. I have also used it for more targeted components in the curriculum. Once I had gained some experience with it as an instructor and saw the energy of group process in learning, and the wonderful fact that I, as the instructor, have the responsibility to design sessions that enable students to apply content rather than just know it, I saw its greater potential: transforming our educational program.

HUNDREDS OF COOKS IN THE KITCHEN COURSE

Let me share with you some specifics on how I adopted TBL for one of our most important courses in the education of our physician's assistants. The course is Introduction to Medicine, spanning two full semesters and using a huge number of guest lecturers who do cameo performances. Some are good, some not. Getting even a handful of the faculty to play from the same music was a challenge. I had no expectation of converting the entire course over to TBL, but I did select a number of key lecture sessions throughout the course to make into TBL sessions.

When replacing a lecture with a TBL session, it was important to keep two points in mind: (a) Reading assignments must sometimes be restructured to more discretely focus on the learning objectives. This was sometimes done by providing the students with a written summary or a couple of relevant journal articles; (b) When students are overloaded with work from other courses, they simply will not take the time to prepare for the TBL session. Know the students, and the competing events in their academic calendar when planning a TBL session.

Because of the success of this, we added more sessions each year. Many of the students welcomed the active mode of what had been a traditional sit-down lecture; some mourned the loss of not being able to do other activities while in a lecture— such as keep up with their e-mail. As my colleagues and I became more skillful with the strategy, the students almost uniformly expressed their appreciation for the new accountability in their learning: preparation for class, working together *very actively* to solve problems, and learning more.

EXAM REVIEW USING TBL

In other courses, I created TBL sessions prior to major exams as powerful review experiences. During the last days before such an exam, almost all students were energized to learn everything they needed to know to do well, and quite anxious about what they felt they did not know. For the TBL review, they came prepared to take a 20–30 question RAT that was graded but not counted. Next, keeping with the TBL protocol, the teams worked on the same set of questions, doing a lot of teaching and learning with one another. Then, they were given a small number of very challenging case study questions as the group application—these questions were very much like the most difficult ones on the upcoming examination. The discussion time provided students plenty of opportunity to fill in their gaps in knowledge

To wind up the TBL review session, students were provided with the opportunity to challenge any of the potential exam items. This often helped to uncover errors, ambiguities, and differences in interpretation that only students seem to be able to find. In some cases a simple grammatical change was all that was needed to improve the item. In other cases, this type of critique caused me to completely throw a question out.

At the end of the exercise the students had gained a little familiarity with my item-writing style, a much better understanding of the objectives, and a big boost in their confidence level. As an added bonus, I had 20 to 30 brand new, piloted test items ready to go into an exam bank for future years.

THE TBL EXAM

We have all, no doubt, observed the posttest hallway behavior of students hungry for immediate feedback from their peers and for confirmation that they made the right choices on a difficult exam. Students also often express a desire to close some knowledge gaps that may have been made painfully evident by an exam. I recognized this as an incredible opportunity for learning.

By slightly modifying some exam procedures, I was able to harness this eagerness to learn. It started by administering the exam in much the same way that we normally administer exams. The students were all provided with a 50-item multiple-choice exam and answer sheet. But, instead of allowing the students to leave the room when they were finished, they were required to remain in their seats until everyone completed the exam.

Once all of the students had completed the individual exam, they grouped into their learning teams to complete the same exam in much the same way that they would complete a group RAT (GRAT). This exercise gave them an opportunity to add extra-credit points to their individual scores based on their team performance. Immediately, I noticed that the discussion of some of the objectives at this point was much more lively, even passionate, than when they completed GRATs in the regular sessions.

On the course evaluations, and in person, the students expressed great satisfaction with the opportunity not only to improve their exam grade, but to go home with a much better understanding of the subject. And, after all, isn't that the point?

THE TBL RADIOLOGY LAB

One of the first experiences that physician assistant students at the University of Florida encountered in their training was gross anatomy. It has always been a demanding course taught at a very quick pace. To facilitate their appreciation of the three-dimensional nature of human anatomy, we offered a supplemental course to gross anatomy called Radiographic Anatomy. This course was a very basic introduction to normal radiographic presentations with a few "abnormals" introduced for contrast.

I have, for a number of years, conducted a student-led laboratory exercise based on a text and a set of plain films by Lucy Frank Squire (1988). The exercise required the students to organize into groups and rotate from one station to the next. Each of the five stations included a programmed text providing historical background and clinical information about the patients in each of the radiographic studies. The texts prompted the students to examine 8 to 10 films at each station and answer some thought-provoking questions. Each team was allowed 30 minutes per station. Over the years, I modified the exercise and introduced CT and MRI studies into the exercise. Students have commented that the exercise was "helpful, but a bit too challenging."

This seemed to be a very natural fit for TBL. I modified the programmed text to include 25 multiple-choice questions very similar to those on a RAT. The questions were distributed throughout the texts so that the teams were challenged to answer five questions at each of the stations.

After consideration of factors such as gender, clinical experience, and grade point average, the students were divided into 10 groups of six. Five groups participated in each of the two 150-minute lab sessions. Each of the groups decided upon a team name and listed it on a scoreboard for all to see. Each of the groups was also provided with an Immediate Feedback-Assessment Technique (IF-AT) response form.

At the end of the exercise, team scores were totaled and posted on the scoreboard and on the class Web site. The team with the winning score was treated to lunch at a local restaurant.

Following the class, students commented that, while the exercise was still very challenging, the structure of the lab activity made the learning more enjoyable and greatly improved their understanding of the topic. It was a definite improvement for their learning and they had more fun.

THE HUMAN PATIENT SIMULATOR

The use of human patient simulators has grown in popularity in a number of medical training programs. Some versions of the machine are quite sophisticated and can provide information such as arterial pressures, vital signs, heart and lung sounds, urine output, and pupil constriction in response to electrical and pharmacologic interventions. With proper planning and programming, detailed algorithms can be constructed to simulate very specific patient scenarios. One of the most important components of successful human patient simulation experiences has been student preparation.

If students show up unprepared, the simulation can get bogged down with discussion of basic concepts. Some educators, by seizing the "teachable moment" in the simulation lab, soon find that time has evaporated before the scenario is complete. The well-prepared students find themselves bored and frustrated by a simulation that has, in effect, stalled while basic principles are explained to the unprepared few.

By presenting the human patient simulation as a dress rehearsal, I found that students took the simulation experience a bit more seriously. This also required me to add preparation experiences that would actively assess their readiness for the simulation. The use of reading assignments followed by individual Readiness Assurance Tests (IRATs) and GRATs was an ideal way to improve their readiness. When preceded by RATs, the human patient simulation then became a group application activity.

One of the courses where I have successfully used TBL with human patient simulation was in an Advanced Cardiac Life Support course. During this course, the students were required to complete four human patient simulations. The simulations were designed to allow students the opportunity to integrate their training in the management of bradycardias, tachycardias, pulseless electrical activity, and asystole. At the beginning of each unit the students were given reading assignments and attended lectures on the appropriate topics. This was followed by IRATs and GRATs of key objectives followed by a human patient simulation session. Each of the teams then participated in a 30-minute simulation.

Each student was put in charge of his or her team for at least 10 minutes. As the scenario unfolded, they were only provided with a few prompts. Each of the exercises was recorded and DVDs were provided to each group to review and critique for their team performance.

MEASURING OUTCOMES

One of the features of TBL that initially appealed to me was the ability to actually document, albeit in an informal way, gains as a result of teamwork. At a number of points during my courses I attempted to measure gains in team performance. This sometimes caused me to reexamine techniques that I used in the classroom or the way that I formed teams. But it also caused me to realize that I could combine this method of measuring gains in team performance with other learning strategies, namely, the group application activity.

In my Advanced Cardiac Life Support course students often walked away from human patient simulations expressing great satisfaction with the experience. But I still wondered how much learning actually occurred compared to the entertainment value provided by the new and innovative technology.

In order to prepare for a simulation session, students were given reading assignments and attended lectures. The simulation sessions were normally preceded by IRATs and GRATs. These assignments and activities required students to arrive well prepared for the simulation exercise.

I found, however, that by scheduling the group RATs after the simulation exercise, I was able to use this as a posttest of sorts. The topic involved the emergent management of tachycardias. My question was whether the teams would perform better on a GRAT following the human patient simulation exercise compared to those teams that had not yet done the simulation.

In this case, the control group (five teams of six), did IRATs and GRATs before the simulation. The experimental group did the IRAT before the simulation and the GRAT afterward. Table 14.1 illustrates the individual and team scores on the RATs. The control group's average score on the IRAT was 76, and the experimental group's average was 72.

At the end of the day, all of the students had demonstrated gains above the average for their team. Figure 14.1 illustrates the gains of the experimental group compared to the control group on RATs. The five teams in the control group demonstrated an average 14% gain over their team averages on the IRAT. The experimental group enjoyed a 26% gain.

These results and my other experiences with TBL have given me a great appreciation for the educational wisdom of TBL. It is a strategy that challenges students to think more deeply about the subject matter at hand because they have to solve real problems, and they learn how to work more collaboratively with their classmates, who will be their colleagues in their profession. For me as an instructor, I have been inspired by the creativity of innovative strategy, and how I have been able to be creative with it. Teaching has become more fun and I feel my students have learned more.

TABLE 14.1
Readiness Assurance Test Scores

Group	Individual Scores			Team Score	Gains		
	Low	High	Mean		vs. Mean	vs. Low	vs. High
Control 1	60	90	75	80	5	20	−10
Control 2	50	100	77	100	23	50	0
Control 3	60	100	77	90	13	30	−10
Control 4	70	100	80	90	10	20	−10
Control 5	50	100	72	90	18	40	−10
All Controls	*50*	*100*	*76*	*90*	*14*	*40*	*−10*
Exp 1	50	80	66	100	34	50	20
Exp 2	50	100	78	90	12	40	−10
Exp 3	40	100	75	100	25	60	0
Exp 4	50	90	73	100	27	50	10
Exp 5	60	80	70	100	30	40	20
All Exp	*40*	*100*	*72*	*98*	*26*	*58*	*−2*

FIGURE 14.1
Team Gains on Readiness Assurance Tests

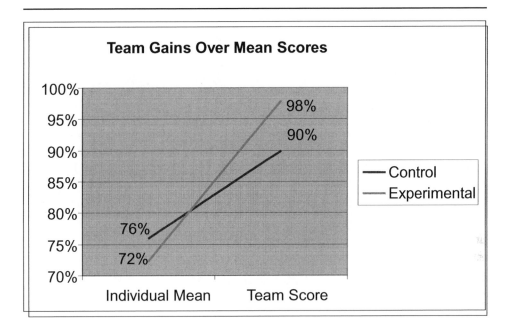

REFERENCE

Squire, L. F. (1988). *Fundamentals of radiology* (4th ed.). Cambridge, MA: Harvard University Press.

CHAPTER 15

The Use of Reading Assignments and Learning Issues as an Alternative to Anatomy Lectures in a Team-Based Learning Curriculum

Nagaswami S. Vasan and David O. DeFouw

We first learned about team-based learning (TBL) when Vasan attended a presentation given by Nancy Searle, of Baylor Medical School, at the Robert Wood Johnson Medical School in the fall of 2003. After the presentation, we discussed TBL and realized its potential to transform the teaching of anatomy by evoking critical thinking in a new clinically integrated approach. We first piloted TBL in the spring of 2004 with our graduate student anatomy program, and then with the summer anatomy program for incoming freshmen medical students and with the concurrent summer enrichment program for upper-level college students taking an advanced anatomy/physiology program.

The students in these programs not only enjoyed the TBL approach but also enthusiastically encouraged us to implement TBL in our first-year anatomy course. Because of the large medical class size and various concerns (see below), we decided to pilot TBL in the anatomy course in the fall of 2004. Over the next year, Vasan attended an Association of American Medical Colleges (AAMC) workshop given by Searle and Dean Parmelee, and he also experienced total immersion in TBL at the Fourth Annual Team-Based Learning Collaborative Conference in Dayton, Ohio, in 2005. In addition, one of the most important resources that has guided us to successfully implement TBL is the book *Team-Based Learning: A Transformative Use of Small Groups in College Teaching* (Michaelsen, Knight, & Fink, 2004).

WHAT LESSONS DID WE LEARN FROM OUR FIRST PILOT STUDY?

- TBL was an excellent substitute for lectures.
- Creating appropriate reading assignments and learning issues to replace lectures was critical.
- Individual Readiness Assurance Tests (IRATs) were essential for each TBL session.

- Group Readiness Assurance Tests (GRATs), where considerable teaching and learning occurs between peers, provided a terrific opportunity for us faculty to clarify any ambiguities and misconceptions.
- TBL required secretarial support.
- TBL fostered deeper learning among the students, and they were excited about coming to class.
- Peer evaluation was meaningful for the students.
- Starting out with a pilot study allowed us to learn the essentials and potential mishaps before expansion.

WHAT QUESTIONS AROSE FROM THE PILOT STUDY?

- Would it work for our very large class sizes (180) and for students with diverse educational backgrounds?
- Is TBL appropriate for a course such as anatomy with an enormous amount of content and a laboratory dissection component?
- Could we really cover all of the material in the same time frame?
- How should we apportion the grade components of TBL in this course?
- Should peer evaluation be graded?
- How will we address the concerns of our fellow faculty and the administration when they learn about the dramatic changes in our teaching format?
- Because of the large class size, do we have the space to conduct simultaneous team encounters without resorting to multiple sessions?

STARTING SMALL

At the New Jersey Medical School (NJMS), gross anatomy has been taught for many, many years using lectures by a host of experienced faculty. We knew that to make a change, we had to have positive outcome data from our pilot to convince others of the viability of TBL in this very traditional course. Coincidentally, in 2004 our undergraduate medical student curriculum was undergoing a reform, so we had a nice window of support to try out TBL with an entire class. This, plus our preliminary findings that the students learned with TBL and were enthusiastic about it, enabled us to present to the various curriculum committees and other basic science departments and move forward.

During the very first week of freshman orientation, we presented an overview of TBL, including the importance of peer evaluation, then conducted a live TBL session based on introductory materials about TBL. The students had their first experience with an IRAT and a GRAT and were ready to go with the upcoming course.

CONCERNS ABOUT COVERING THE COURSE CONTENT

In a course like anatomy with a vast amount of content traditionally taught by a team of research-oriented basic scientists, there is resistance to making any significant changes in how the course is taught. Lectures are seen as efficient and economical ways to teach, especially in comparison to small-group teaching, and making any change is likely to take considerable time and energy on the part of a faculty already stretched for time. The greatest fear of our colleagues was that we could not cover the same amount of content with this method, therefore our students might know less. We were not as concerned about this because of the successes of others in similar courses elsewhere (Dinan, 2004; Nieder, Parmelee, Stolfi, & Hudes, 2005). In fact, we felt strongly that the approach would take care of the content plus help our students better apply what they learned.

OUR COURSE—GROSS ANATOMY—WHAT WE DID

Encouraged by the successes of TBL in other science courses, our own experiences with it in the pilot ventures, and feeling ready to transform "the sage on the stage" entrenchment of lecture-based instruction to our faculty, becoming a "guide on the side" (Herreid, 1998), we wanted to expand TBL. In addition, as we all have learned over the past 10–15 years, students are attending lectures in declining numbers. Many come out of guilt and/or to be with their friends for a part of the day. How much they actually learn via lectures has become an increasing question as we stand at a podium, with PowerPoint behind us and a half-empty lecture hall before us. Contrary to our long-held beliefs about the learning in lectures, students who do not come always seem to do just fine on exams.

Our gross anatomy course is offered over an 18–19 week period and is divided into three units: thorax, back, and upper extremity (6 weeks), head and neck (5 weeks), and abdomen, pelvis, perineum, and lower extremity (7–8 weeks). There are three unit exams and two mid-unit mini exams, which contain embryology questions based on embryology lectures given to the entire class, and anatomy questions that had been derived from the lectures. But, with TBL, we changed these to come from the reading assignments and "learning issues" (see below). For the graded written exams, students receive both an individual grade (IRAT) and a group grade (GRAT). The GRAT amounts to 15% of the final course grade. An important process of our TBL is that if a team successfully challenges a question, all the teams receive credit for that question. We also have three individually graded lab practical exams (30% of the final grade) that correspond to the contents of the three unit exams. The individual exam scores represent 85%, which is a very high percentage for individual work within the TBL strategy. We conduct peer evaluations after each unit exam, but they do not contribute to the final grade.

Starting with the 2004 academic year, we eliminated lectures for the course and developed specific reading assignments and learning issues for the students to master prior to coming to class. The learning issues focused on the material relevant to clinical anatomy enabling the students to solve clinical problems in the subject. We created an ungraded IRAT of five to seven questions for each weekly TBL session, but we scored these immediately so that students knew how well they had prepared.

At this point, we did provide focused instruction on the concepts covered in the IRAT, then the teams were administered the GRAT, scored immediately with an Immediate Feedback-Assessment Technique (IF-AT) form.

Even without counting the weekly IRATs, we had 100% class attendance for these sessions! The combination of having an opportunity to answer questions on their out-of-class assignments *and* to work with their teammates on the same questions was a terrific motivator. The reading assignments included lists of pages from the text to either study or omit, points of clinical relevance, concepts to be developed, and resources to use. They used the learning issues effectively to focus on the relevant clinical anatomy and became intensely engaged in clinical reasoning as they solved the problems posed in our questions. Students were not inhibited to ask for peer explanation of difficult concepts. The students learned more than specific anatomical knowledge, and they used many resources to expand their fund of clinically relevant knowledge. The atmosphere was positive, built student trust in one another, improved communication skills, and helped to develop good interpersonal relationships. Sessions lasted 90 minutes, and we tailored the numbers and difficulty of questions to fit, based upon some of our pilot experiences of the previous summer and spring.

The TBL that we implemented diverges from the classic approach described by Michaelsen and others (2004), and practiced by others. Except for the five TBL encounters that follow the exams (individual and team grades were recorded), the weekly team encounters with IRAT and GRAT were not graded. Each question in the IRAT, whether graded or not, was case-based requiring students to apply what they were learning. Hence, we have not included a separate phase three (application of course concepts) as described in the classic TBL approaches.

Because of the large class size (180 students), the TBL sessions were held in the anatomy dissection lab. The two authors floated throughout the class during team discussion of learning issues and when necessary provided explanations. During freshman orientation of the 2006 academic year, a group of enthusiastic second-year students composed and showed a video of "good, bad and ugly teams" to emphasize the best practices and behaviors in team-based learning. The first-year students were highly impressed by the video, and it served as a powerful tool to shape their appreciation of TBL from the onset of the course.

Our freshmen class typically consists of about 10% of students in the seven-year program (three years undergraduate and four years medical school) and 30%–35% of students with postgraduate education and/or work/life experiences. We created the teams by using the student academic profiles so that each team was balanced in males/females, similar education and experience, and ethic background. Interestingly, professors of other courses with the same students use the same teams for their small-group interaction.

We elected to not have peer evaluation contribute to the course grades. We did, however, keep track of the peer evaluation scores (see Appendix 15.A) and provided proactive counseling to the very few students who were consistently getting low scores from their peers. As expected, these same students were invariably getting the lowest grades in the class already—in large part, we believe, because of their lack of proper preparation for class. Students who received exemplary scores from their peers were almost always at the top of the class in their grades, and we used this information at the next year's freshman orientation to emphasize the importance of preparation and working collaboratively to make the team successful.

OUR OUTCOMES FOR TBL IN GROSS ANATOMY

Academic

The performance on departmental exams shows that students in the TBL curriculum tended to perform better than the students in the traditional curriculum (Table 15.1). It is possible that TBL improved students' preparedness by keeping up with the assignments and not by cramming before exams. Furthermore, the peer pressure to contribute to team discussions and share resources contributed to their enhanced performance.

In addition to the expected benefits to learning for students through TBL, a number of factors might have contributed to the improved performance on the National Board of Medical Examiners (NBME) subject exam. These include (a) the inclusion of clinical application exercises for discussion during team encounters, (b) the improved quality of unit exam questions written in collaboration with clinical faculty, and (b) incorporation of high-quality problem-solving and clinical reasoning questions obtained from various sources in our TBL discussions.

Student Opinion

Fresh out of college, many students had initial reactions such as, "What! No anatomy lectures?" That exclamation rapidly changed after one or two TBL sessions

TABLE 15.1
Summary of Student Performances in the Traditional Versus TBL Curriculum

Types of Curriculum	Examinations			
	Unit 1	Unit 2	Unit 3	NBME
2002 (Traditional)	79	81	79	70
2003 (Traditional)	70	73	77	64
2004 (TBL)	77	81	80	72
2005 (TBL)	81	88	85	72
GRAT (2005)	97	98	97	

Note. This table summarizes student performances in the traditional versus TBL curriculum. Class averages for individual exams are listed.

as students experienced how team cohesiveness evolved rapidly and how the interactive process expanded their thinking and processing for deeper learning. Here are some typical comments: "TBL is the best instructive tool at NJMS. Love TBL, and its involvement in our learning"; "The TBL process is extraordinarily helpful"; "The TBL components are one of the most effective means of learning"; "TBLs!!! All courses should be taught using TBLs!" and "TBL keeps students up to date on readings."

CONCLUSIONS AND RECOMMENDATIONS

Our medical school's new curriculum in 2004 included a reduction in the time provided for our course in gross anatomy. Also, at the same time a number of our core faculty departed, leaving us two as the principle teachers for the whole course. Luckily, we had TBL as an option to help provide the students with a course that would equip them with the knowledge to proceed with their professions. As you can see, their academic performance improved with these changes, and we feel it did so as a result of TBL. With continued refinement of team assignments and additional clinical application cases for TBL discussion, we anticipate that students might better retain their knowledge of anatomy for application to their clerkship years and beyond.

From the pilot work we did and from experiencing the excitement of our students, Vasan was inspired to apply to become a Harvard Macy Scholar, using TBL in gross anatomy as his project. The Harvard Macy Scholar Program is the preeminent faculty development program for aspiring leaders in innovation in medical education. He was selected in 2006, shared his experiences with an illustrious group of other teaching scholars, and in 2007 was invited to be one of the program's faculty scholars.

We highly recommend that faculty interested in TBL read about it from the growing list of peer-reviewed journal articles, the books about TBL like this one, attend the annual Team-Based Learning Collaborative Conference that has training workshops, and join the Team-Based Learning Collaborative.

REFERENCES

Dinan, F. J. (2004). An alternative to lecturing in the sciences. In L. K. Michaelsen, A. B. Knight, & L. D. Fink (Eds.), *Team-based learning: A transformative use of small groups in college teaching* (pp. 97–104). Sterling, VA: Stylus.

Herreid, C. F. (1998). Why isn't cooperative learning used to teach science? *Bioscience 48,* 553–559.

Michaelsen, L. K., Knight, A. B., & Fink, L. D. (Eds.). (2004). *Team-based learning: A transformative use of small groups in college teaching*. Sterling, VA: Stylus.

Nieder, G. L., Parmelee, D. X., Stolfi, A., & Hudes, P. D. (2005). Team-based learning in a medical gross anatomy and embryology course. *Clinical Anatomy, 18,* 56–63.

APPENDIX 15.A

Team-Based Learning Peer Evaluation

TEAM

Student Name		Punctuality	Preparedness	Contribution	Respect	Flexibility

Rankings:
5: Strongly agree **4**: To a large extent agree **3**: Agree **2**: Disagree; **1**: Strongly disagree

Punctuality: Came to team activities on time and stayed until the end.
Preparedness: Came prepared for team activities.
Contribution: Contributed to team discussions.
Respect for others: Encouraged others to contribute.
Flexibility: Considered different points of view.

- -

Feedback on Team Process:

1. List ways in which members of your team contributed to the creation of a positive learning environment, and identify those members who are particularly good at each of the (above) listed behaviors.
2. What could members of your team do that would help most to improve your team's performance?

CHAPTER 16

Team-Based Learning in
Sport and Exercise Psychology

Case Studies and Concept Maps as Application Exercises

Karla A. Kubitz

I was ripe for a change in teaching strategy when I came across Harry Meeuwsen's (2003) article on team-based learning (TBL) in the *North American Society for the Psychology of Sport and Physical Activity Newsletter*. I was primarily a traditional teacher/lecturer, equipped with PowerPoint slides and printed handouts, and I'd had a particularly unpleasant semester, one in which my students seemed to hate almost everything I did in the classroom. Consequently, I was intrigued by Meeuwsen's description of the TBL strategy and of how it had revitalized his teaching and increased student learning and student engagement. In order to find out more about the strategy, I visited Larry Michaelsen's TBL Web site http://www.ou.edu/idp/teamlearning/ and I read the Michaelsen, Knight, and Fink (2004) book.

Despite some trepidation, I decided to try TBL in an upcoming minimester class (i.e., a condensed class offered over the three-week winter break). I had a really good experience in that class and have been hooked on TBL ever since. I no longer struggle with how many slides to make or how to keep my students awake as I work my way through them. Instead, I teach all of my courses, about eight a year, as TBL courses. In this chapter, I will describe my implementation of TBL (including the way that I use case studies and concept maps in application exercises) and the impact that it has had on me and on my students. I will also present some suggestions, drawn from my experiences, for those considering implementing TBL in their classes.

My classes include all the traditional components of TBL. That is, sometime during the first week or so of class, I assign students, as heterogeneously as possible, to teams, and the students remain with (and do much of their work with) their teams throughout the semester. Although the numbers vary from semester to semester, I typically have five teams per class with five to seven students per team. Each team chooses a team name and has a team folder for tracking attendance and performance. I also take a team picture to help us all learn each other's names. In addition, as is traditional, my classes include individual Readiness Assurance Tests (IRATs), group Readiness Assurance Tests (GRATs), appeals, and simple, as well as increasingly

complex, individual and team application exercises. Finally, individual and team performance, as well as team maintenance (as determined by peer evaluation), count as
part of the course grade (i.e., typically in a 60/30/10 individual/team/team maintenance ratio).

I normally have nine RATs during a semester and each 12-question RAT covers
one to two chapters from the textbook (see Appendix 16.A). Each RAT contains a
mix of knowledge, comprehension, and application level (Fink, 2003) questions, and
I provide a test blueprint, a set of 13–15 learning objectives to guide the students'
study efforts (see Appendix 16.B). I also allow students to bring in one page of
handwritten notes to use during the RATs.[1] Students take their IRATs first, noting
their choices on a Scantron form and on the RAT itself, and when done, they put
their completed Scantrons in their team folder. When all the Scantrons have been
turned in, team folders are brought to me. When all the team folders have been
brought to me, students gather with their teammates to take their GRAT. They use
the Immediate Feedback-Assessment Technique (IF-AT) form during the GRAT. In
doing so, they receive immediate feedback about their choices. Moreover, students
are allowed to indicate two possible answers for each of the questions on the IRAT
and GRAT and, consequently, to receive credit for partial knowledge.

Finally, after concluding the GRAT, I provide a mini lecture or lead a focused
conversation (i.e., a purposeful, guided discussion that flows from objective to reflective to interpretive to decisional questions; Stanfield, 2000) about the RAT/reading
material (see Appendix 16.C).

Once the students have gained their initial exposure to the course material via the
RAT, the next task in traditional TBL is to involve them in using it to solve real-
world, course-relevant problems through application exercises. In terms of application exercises, I include individual and team as well as topic-specific and integrative
exercises. Individual application exercises are done prior to and in preparation for
team application exercises. Topic-specific application exercises occur during the
classes subsequent to a RAT and focus on the material from the most recent RAT
(see Appendix 16.D). Integrative Application Exercises (IAEs) occur three to four
times a semester and integrate material from several RATs. Preclass preparation is
encouraged by requiring an individual IAE (see Appendix 16.E) to be submitted
(online) at least two hours prior to the team IAE (see Appendix 16.F). The final
exam, is a fourth, individual IAE and it allows the students to demonstrate the
cumulative effect of having completed (and received feedback on) previous IAEs.

One of my biggest TBL-related challenges was constructing application exercises,
particularly psychological-content-based exercises, that would meet Michaelsen and
others' (2004) same problem, specific choice, and simultaneous reporting criteria. In
the end, I combined Meeuwsen's (2003) poster assignment with concept mapping.
For those who might be unfamiliar with the term, concept mapping is a learning
technique that helps students visually organize their knowledge of a subject
(Novak & Gowin, 1996). Moreover, concept mapping develops critical thinking
skills because students have to decide which ideas to include in a map and how to
depict the interrelationships among their ideas. I focus the concept mapping assignments on different types of case studies, including those drawn from case study

books, from psychologically themed movies, or from course-related current events, and I provide team whiteboards (MacIsaac, 2004) for use in concept mapping exercises.[2]

In my exercise psychology class, the topic-specific and integrative application exercises focus on the competitors in the 2004 *Discovery Health Channel's National Body Challenge*, a televised eight-week national fitness and weight-loss challenge. Topic-specific application exercises require creating a concept map that illustrates the application of one theory or model to a competitor's problem (see Appendix 16.D). IAEs require creating concept maps that illustrate the application of multiple theories or models to a competitor's problem (see Appendix 16.E and Appendix 16.F). Simpler integrative assignments (given earlier in the semester) require depicting only causes and solutions of a competitor's problem. More complex assignments (given later in the semester) require a more sophisticated approach and may focus on the competitor and his or her personal trainer.

Teams work together on their team maps over the course of one or two class periods (depending on the length of the class period). When they have completed their work, they post their maps (simultaneously and anonymously) on the walls of the classroom (see Appendix 16.H and Appendix 16.I) for critiquing. Posted maps typically include one or two instructor-created maps, designed to stimulate discussion—these may even portray incorrect information to inspire debate. Individuals examine and critique the maps, attempting to identify scientifically defensible kudos, namely, correct application of course material, and kvetches, namely, incorrect application of course material. Teams pool their ideas, select their best kudo and kvetch, write them on Post-it notes, and post them (simultaneously) on the appropriate maps. Teams then examine their feedback (i.e., the kudos and kvetches for their map) and use it to critique their own maps (see Appendix 16.G). Finally, all students describe what they learned and how they learned it in a "Minute" paper (see Appendix 16.J).

As is traditional in TBL, students in my classes evaluate each other's team maintenance, that is, their contributions to team performance. I use Michaelsen and others' (2004, p. 266) version of peer evaluation. This means that at the end of the semester students complete a Team Maintenance Evaluation in which they award an average of 10 points per person to each of their team members. They are asked to discriminate some in their ratings, giving at least one 9 and one 11 and to provide an explanation for their highest and lowest ratings. I then calculate a team maintenance score for each person from the averaged peer evaluations for each team. I ask that the students sit separately from their teammates when they complete the Team Maintenance Evaluation, and that they sign a statement saying that they have provided an honest assessment of their teammates' contributions, that is, one not based on an in- or out-of-class agreement to distribute points in a way that does not take individual effort into account.

TBL has benefited my students and me. I have benefited in two ways. First, I have a clearer sense of what I want my students to be able to do when they have completed my classes. I want them to be able to apply psychological theories and models in their work with real people in the real world. Both my RATs and my application exercises are designed with this outcome in mind. I also have a better understanding of the challenges that psychological theories and models pose for students. Quite often, students see familiar words, like *achievement* and *goal* and think that they already know achievement goal theory. Conversely, they see depictions of psychological models, with their plethora of constructs, boxes, and interconnecting arrows, and are so intimidated that they don't even try to understand what the models represent. Knowing this helps me design application exercises that challenge and scaffold (support) their learning.

Second, I have a radically different role in the classroom, having moved from "sage on the stage" to "guide on the side" (King, 1993). This means that I no longer deliver course material, neatly packaged as slides and handouts. Instead, I facilitate the student's acquisition of the course material. In fact, when TBL is really working for me, it feels like the students and I are working *together* on the goal of learning to apply the course material.

At the end of the semester, I hold a focused conversation with my students about their experiences in my course (see Appendix 16.K). The following comments come from these conversations. I find that students *can* identify specific theories or models that they have learned during the semester. They tell me that they learned these things through reading the course material, through taking notes for the RATs, through discussing the material with their teammates, through creating concept maps, and through applying the course material to the Body Challenge competitors or other case studies.

They often emphasize that the repetition inherent in TBL keeps the course material in their minds throughout the semester. Most students seem to feel that the course material was interesting and will be useful to them in the real world. Although there are exceptions,[3] the majority of students feel positive about how and what they learned. They tell me that they enjoyed the team activities, that watching the Body Challenge episodes helped make the course material "come alive," and that having to draw concept maps clarified their understanding of the course material. Most of the students also tell me that they learned more and enjoyed the class more than if it had been taught in the traditional way. They say that they probably would have been bored or put to sleep by lectures and that doing a variety of activities in class made coming to class easier. This sentiment is particularly strong in my longer classes (e.g., the three-hour minimester or Friday afternoon classes).

Students tell me that they have changed in various ways as a result of my class. They say that they have improved their ability to work with others, speaking up in the classroom, managing time, and reading more of the assigned textbooks. Finally, students have made many good suggestions for improving the course, including (a) make assignments available earlier; (b) be more specific about what is required for an application exercise; (c) provide more instruction and assistance with concept mapping; (d) vary the types of application exercises, for example, fewer concept mapping assignments; (e) convert the 50-minute class into a longer one. They would also like to have the final exam in the form of a team assignment!

In this chapter, I have described my implementation of TBL and the impact that it has had on me and on my students. I would like to close by presenting some suggestions, drawn from my experiences, for those considering implementing this strategy in their classes. First, tightly knit the key components, learning goals and objectives, the RATs, and the application exercises. That is, make sure that learning goals and objectives are reflected in test blueprints, *and* that test blueprint items are matched with RAT questions, *and* that RAT questions are expanded upon in application exercises. Following Michaelsen and others' (2004) getting started guidelines and identifying "doing" objectives will make it easier to design a tightly interwoven TBL class. Second, write *good* multiple-choice questions, particularly questions that assess higher levels of thinking. Questions that assess higher levels of thinking will create lively intrateam discussions during GRATs. I have found Haladyna's (1994, 1997) books on writing multiple-choice questions incredibly helpful in this endeavor. Third, take advantage of the knowledge of the other members of the TBL community. In person and via e-mail, they have helped me to improve my courses, and much of my success with TBL is the direct result of their feedback and suggestions.

NOTES

1. I've recently begun asking students who don't bring in a sheet of handwritten notes to sign a statement acknowledging their "seeming" lack of preparation and accepting the consequences of this oversight for their course grade. Doing so seems to have decreased the number of students without handwritten notes.

2. My whiteboards are pieces of white tile board (32 inches wide and 24 inches long) that can be written on with dry erase markers during team assignments. Teams place the whiteboard in the center of their pushed-together tables (or on top of several pushed-together desks) and can then brainstorm more easily. When they're ready, whiteboards can be displayed around the room by leaning them against the walls, standing them on the edges of chalkboards/whiteboards, or by having students hold them up.

3. Those who are less positive about their experience in my class tell me that they didn't like TBL because they felt like they were "teaching themselves" and that they would have preferred for me to lecture because it's easier on them (that is, because they don't have to prepare for class) and because it's more familiar to them.

REFERENCES

Fink, D. (2003). *Creating significant learning experiences: An integrated approach to designing college courses.* San Francisco: Josey-Bass.

Haladyna, T. M. (1994). *Developing and validating multiple-choice test items.* Hillsdale, NJ: Lawrence Erlbaum.

Haladyna, T. M. (1997). *Writing test items to evaluate higher order thinking.* Needham Heights, MA: Allyn & Bacon.

Hollander, E. (1967). *Principles and methods of social psychology*. Oxford, UK: Oxford University Press.

King, A. (1993). From sage on the stage to guide on the side. *College Teaching, 41*, 30–35.

MacIsaac, D. (2004). *Whiteboarding in the classroom*. Retrieved from http://physicsed.buffalo state.edu/AZTEC/BP_WB/

Meeuwsen, H. (2003, Fall). Changing your students' learning: From apathy to engagement. *North American Society for the Psychology of Sports and Physical Activity, 28*, 10–11.

Michaelsen, L. K., Knight, A. B., & Fink, L. D. (2004). *Team-based learning: A transformative use of small groups in college teaching*. Sterling, VA: Stylus.

Novak, J. D., & Gowin, D. B. (1996). *Learning how to learn*. New York: Cambridge University Press.

Stanfield, R. B. (Ed.). (2000). *The art of focused conversation*. Gabriola Island, B.C., Canada: New Society Publishers.

APPENDIX 16.A

Sample RAT

Name: _____

Instructions: Each question on the RAT is potentially worth two points (i.e., 24 pts total). Depending on your level of confidence/preparation, do one of the following: (a) choose one best answer and enter it on *two* consecutive lines on the Scantron. If your choice is correct, you will earn two points; *or* (b) choose two answers that you think are equally likely and enter them in *two* consecutive spaces on the Scantron. If at least one of your choices is correct, you will earn one point.

1/1–2/1

George went for a 20-min run after class. Which is the best descriptor?
   a. acute exercise
   b. chronic exercise
   c. anaerobic exercise
   d. exercise adherence

2/3–4/3

Which of the following is *not* one of the Healthy People 2010 physical activity and fitness objectives?
   a. decreasing inactive leisure activity
   b. increasing worksite fitness programs
   c. increasing daily physical education
   d. increasing adolescent activity
   e. decreasing television watching

12/11–12/12

Which of the following exemplifies a physical activity epidemiology study?
   a. The study examines the effects of doctor's advice on physical activity levels.
   b. The study examines physical activity levels in the population by surveying people at the mall.
   c. The study examines the effects of music on perceived exertion during exercise.
   d. The study examines the relationship between actual and self-reported physical activity.
   e. The study examines the effects of physical fitness on self-esteem.

Note: The numbering scheme on the RAT helps keep the students on track when using the split-point format. The first number on the left is the question number. The pair of numbers in the middle are the lines that should be filled in on the Scantron form. The third number at the right is the line to be scratched off on the IF-AT form.

APPENDIX 16.B

Sample Test Blueprint

Test Blueprint/RAT #1 (Ch. 1 & 2)

	In order to be prepared for the RAT, please be sure that you:
1	can distinguish acute and chronic exercise, and adoption and adherence.
2	recognize the Healthy People 2010 physical activity and fitness objectives.
3	can identify a physical activity epidemiology study.

Note: There is a close conceptual match between the items on the Test Blueprint and the related questions on the RAT.

APPENDIX 16.C

Sample Post-RAT Focused Conversation Questions

The focused conversation technique, described by Stanfeld (2000) is a purposeful, guided discussion technique. During a focused conversation, students are guided through four types of questions. More specifically, in a focused conversation, questioning proceeds from objective (O) to reflective (R) to interpretive (I) to decisional (D) types of questions. The questions below follow Stanfield's ORID framework.

Objective
   What did you learn today?

Reflective
   What was familiar?
   What was surprising?
   What was confusing?

Interpretive
   How does this information relate to what you already know?
   What's missing from this material?

Decisional
   How will you apply what you learned?

APPENDIX 16.D

Sample Topic-Specific Application Exercise

1. Review your notes on Todd, from the *Discovery Health Channel's National Body Challenge* DVD.

2. Complete the concept map below illustrating Hollander's (1967) model of personality (including the model's three levels) and classifying a sampling of Todd's personality characteristics, that is, at least three per level according to level.

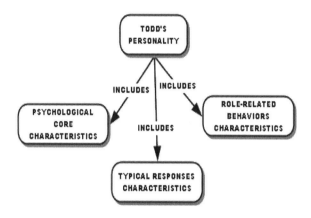

APPENDIX 16.E

Sample *Individual* Integrative Application Exercise

This assignment will help prepare you for the Team Integrative Application Exercise to be done in class. Please download the file and follow the instructions to complete the assignment. You may use your book and/or notes. However, please complete the assignment without assistance of others. When you have completed the assignment, do *three* things.

1. Submit the assignment online at least *two* hours before class.
2. Print a hard copy of the assignment and bring it to class.
3. Sign the statement below.

- -

I completed this assignment myself and did not copy it from a fellow student.

Name: _____

Date: _____

1. Review your notes about the participants in the *Discovery Health Channel's National Body Challenge* DVD. In the *Body Challenge*, Algie has a serious problem. That is, he is sedentary.
2. Using what you've learned thus far this semester, identify the scientifically defensible "causes of" and potential "solutions for" Algie's problem. You may use your book and/or your notes as you work, and you should try to apply the theories and models of exercise psychology that we have been focusing on in the RATs and the topic specific assignments.
3. Create a concept map illustrating your thoughts about Algie's problem, its causes, and potential solutions. You should use concept mapping software (e.g., Inspiration, C-map, etc.) to create your map. Organize your map so that the problem (Algie's sedentary behavior) is in the middle, the causes are on the left, and the solutions are on the right.

APPENDIX 16.F

Sample *Team* Integrative Application Exercise

1. This assignment focuses on Algie from the *Discovery Health Channel's National Body Challenge* DVD. Algie has a serious problem. That is, Algie is sedentary. You are to create a team concept map depicting scientifically defensible causes and solutions for Algie's problem. Maps will be evaluated using the grading rubric below.

Grading Rubric

Above average: The map demonstrated exemplary use of the course material. That is, the map included a very well-thought-out selection of course material. In addition, the course material was always used correctly and with considerable depth of understanding. Moreover, the map was extraordinarily carefully drawn and unusually thoughtfully labeled.

Average: The map demonstrated competent use of the course material. That is, the map included a rather well-thought-out selection of course material. In addition, the course material was mostly used correctly and with some depth of understanding. Moreover, the map was carefully drawn and thoughtfully labeled.

Below Average: The map demonstrated emerging use of the course material. That is, the map included relatively little course material. In addition, the course material may have been used either incorrectly or superficially much of the time and the map may have not have been carefully drawn and/or carefully labeled.

---

2. Begin your work by sharing the scientifically defensible causes and solutions for Algie's problem that you identified in your preclass Individual Integrative Assignments. Create a draft version, bringing your ideas together, of your team concept map using the whiteboards and dry erase markers. Organize it so that "Algie's sedentary behavior" is in the middle, the causes are on the left side, and the solutions are on the right side.

3. Create a final version of your team map using the chart paper and permanent markers. Write as neatly as possible and large enough so that someone looking at your map from afar will be able to read it. In addition, please write a one-page narrative that puts your map into words. When you are finished, write your team name on the back of your map and narrative in pencil and turn them in to me.

4. When all teams are finished working, I will post the team maps (and also one or more maps that I created) on the walls of the classroom and you will critique the posted maps, attempting to identify scientifically defensible kudos and kvetches. Kudos are praiseworthy aspects and kvetches are problematic aspects of the maps.

5. After you have critiqued the maps, you will share your potential kudos and kvetches with your teammates and pick a single best kudo and best kvetch to write up on a Post-it. When all teams are ready, kudos and kvetches will be posted on the maps. Kudos and kvetches based on scientifically defensible issues will be worth 3 bonus points each.

6. When the kudos and kvetches have been posted, you will evaluate your own team maps and your team processes using the team self-evaluation form and you will also assess your individual learning via a "Minute" paper.

APPENDIX 16.G

Sample Team Self-Evaluation Form

Team Name: _____

I. Answer the questions below.
    1. Which poster did your team think was the best poster (aside from your own)? Why?
    2. Did your team map receive any kudos? If so, what were they for?
    3. Did your team map receive any kvetches? If so, what were they for? Were they valid? Why? Why not?
    4. What things did you as a team do well this time?
    5. What things do you plan to do differently or better next time?
    6. What things could the instructor do to help your team perform better next time?

II. Apply the grading rubric to your poster. Circle your decision and explain your rationale below.

Above Average . . . . Average . . . . Below Average

Rationale:

APPENDIX 16.H

Sample Team Map #1 (see Inspiration Software)

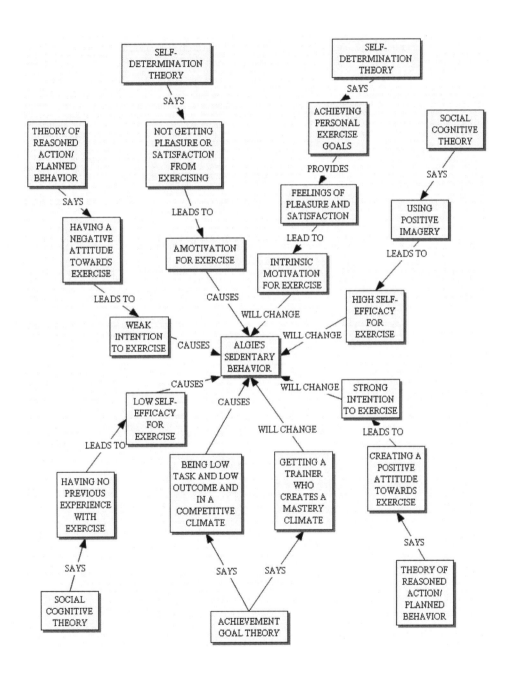

APPENDIX 16.I

Sample Team Map #2 (see Inspiration Software)

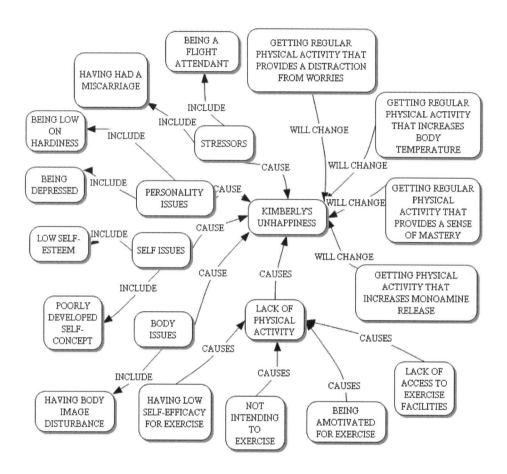

APPENDIX 16.J

Excerpts from Minute Papers

Minute papers were completed at the end of the team integrative assignments. Students were instructed to write for about a minute on the following question.

What did you learn from the integrative assignment and how did you learn it?

- I learned to be more prepared for class and to take people's suggestions to make my map more complete.
- I learned that it is a lot better when a group of people put all their ideas into one, and then a larger group of people critiques them. It helps you see your strengths and understand your mistakes.
- I learned that sometimes your group can make mistakes, but it doesn't matter as long as everyone shares responsibility for the mistake. This is what my team did.
- I learned that, when coming together as a team, many more ideas are brought to the table. For example, other team members remembered things about Kimberly that I didn't. I think we have become more interactive as a team and it has helped us to excel in the team assignments.
- I learned that if I think something on our poster is wrong, I should stand by my opinion and use the book to verify what is correct.
- I learned that, even as a group, we can be wrong. We mixed up Type A and Type B. The other groups picked up on that. It was also good to see that some of the things we had on our paper were the same as the things on the other groups' papers. It made us feel like we had learned something.
- I learned about the options I never thought about before. I don't think in such great detail, but by looking at other teams' concept maps, I was able to see what we missed and how we assessed the question differently. It kind of opened our minds to a different level. It was very helpful to see the differences.
- I learned how to correctly apply theories and models. It was helpful to discuss information with my group to gain a better understanding on how to apply theories. Posting kudos and kvetches made me focus on what theories were correctly used. Being able to see what other people posted helped our team realize we could have put in more information.
- From this team assignment, I learned that by splitting up the work on the benefits and causes of Kimberly being unhappy, we finished faster, but instead of having all seven team members giving their ideas on each topic, we only had three people doing that. The others were working on the benefits from physical activity. Next time, we should go through the map as a group to come up with as many options as possible.
- I learned that working as a team is better than working as an individual because we all had great ideas as well as some that were wrong. It was good to help each other and come up with a good concept map together.

APPENDIX 16.K

End-of-the-Semester Focused Conversation Questions

Objective Questions
>   What specific information or ideas have you learned this semester?
>   How did you learn these things?

Reflective Questions
>   How do you feel about what you learned?
>   How do you feel about *how* you learned?

Interpretive Questions
>   Compared to how much you would have learned, if this course had been taught
>   in the "traditional" way, how much did you learn?
>   Compared to how much you would have enjoyed it, if the course had been taught
>   in the "traditional" way, how much did you enjoy it?

Decisional Questions
>   How have you changed as a result of this course?
>   If you could have changed anything about the course, what would it have been?

CHAPTER 17

Team-Based Learning in a Psychiatry Clerkship

Cheryl S. Al-Mateen

At most medical schools, the third year is devoted to clerkship experiences in which students are assigned to the core areas of medicine for varying amounts of time. On these clerkships, students are expected to evaluate many patients under the supervision of residents and faculty, and across the year they are given increasing amounts of responsibility in the care and management of patients. During this formative year, students learn how to perform the many basic procedures in medicine and surgery, for example, venipuncture, suturing, starting IV lines, and how to present the cases they evaluate succinctly and coherently to their supervisors and clinical care teams. It is in this year that medical students start to apply the basic medical science information they have learned over the previous two years.

I became the director of our psychiatry clerkship in July 2004 and conducted a needs assessment. There had been few changes in the experience for students in many years. I met with the chair, the director of Undergraduate Psychiatry Education, clerkship faculty, and reviewed student evaluations. I explored how the psychiatry clerkship is conducted at other medical schools and wrote a review of ours to share with the chair and faculty. Fortunately, the chair of the Department of Psychiatry and the director of Undergraduate Psychiatry Education were supportive of innovations to enhance student learning. Team-based learning (TBL) was instituted in August 2005 on both of the Virginia Commonwealth University (VCU) School of Medicine campuses; the Medical College of Virginia campus in Richmond, and the INOVA Health System campus in Fairfax, which had just begun training students on their psychiatry clerkship.

How were our students spending their time? Students were spending four and one-half days each week on a clinical service for six weeks, with one-half day weekly devoted to didactic sessions conducted by the faculty. In Richmond, there were seven different clinical sites, four on our campus. All students participated in a rotational on-call duty at our main hospital. Our clinical sites included a large forensic state hospital, a community mental health center, the department's outpatient clinic, a Veterans Administration hospital, a child and adolescent psychiatric hospital, inpatient wards, and the consultation and liaison service in the main hospital.

From the needs assessment, it was clear that the students were getting an excellent set of clinical experiences. However, they were not reading the core content for the clerkship. They were reading review books and board prep question books to prepare for the required end-of-clerkship nationally standardized exam. We were concerned that their education in psychiatry was without the appropriate depth to comprehensively understand and care for patients, regardless of what specialty they would eventually enter. The didactic portion of the clerkship consisted of lectures by faculty on a range of topics; some of the faculty were good at involving the students in an interactive learning experience, but other sessions were "dry" according to student evaluation.

I reviewed the literature on adult learning theory to confirm what I knew: active and student-centered approaches are the most effective means to enhance learning (Arseneau & Rodenburg, 1998; Guild & Garger, 1998; Kaufman, 2003). The use of such methods increases student enthusiasm, the amount of material that is learned and retained, and promotes lifelong learning (Arseneau & Rodenburg, 1998). The literature also shows that assessment of learning should be conducted in a variety of ways, not just focusing on the facts learned, but also on how the knowledge is applied in the clinical context, for example, clinician performance in vitro and in vivo (Wass, van der Vleuten, Shatzer, & Jones, 2001).

Medical education has embraced these approaches, and there has been a focus on learner-centered education at some of the preeminent institutions (Armstrong, 1997). A curriculum should include a variety of teaching approaches because of the different learning styles among our students (Guild & Garger, 1998; Kern, Thomas, Howard, & Bass, 1998). Discussion, problem-based learning, simulations, and learning projects by individuals and groups are encouraged (Kern et al., 1998). Learning projects are key to successful problem-based learning (PBL) and the newer TBL. Many schools use PBL as the central instructional mode for the basic medical sciences curriculum, and it appears to work well (Hoffman & Headrick, 2006). TBL has more recently begun to be used in medical schools' basic medical science curricula.

We invited Ruth Levine, who had started to use TBL in her psychiatry clerkship at the University of Texas Medical Branch (UTMB) at Galveston, to conduct a workshop on how she had implemented the strategy. She was the first to publish a peer-reviewed article on the use of TBL in a clerkship (Levine et al., 2004), and is a nationally known consultant for the strategy. She worked with our faculty in a full-day workshop, and we have now created several TBL modules covering key topic areas in psychiatry (see Table 17.1).

IMPLEMENTATION

My faculty and I elected to follow the prescribed protocol for TBL (Michaelsen, 2004). Therefore, we have developed specific objectives (see Table 17.2), reading assignments to be completed before each session, individual Readiness Assurance Tests (IRATs), the group Readiness Assurance Test (GRAT), application exercises, and peer evaluation. TBL counts for 15% of the final grade in the psychiatry clerkship. The reading assignment for the orientation session includes an introduction to

TABLE 17.1
Didactic Sessions

Original Didactic Sessions	New Didactic Series TBL* Format
Orientation	*Orientation
Psychopharmacology	*Psychopharmacology
Schizophrenia and psychotic disorders	*The psychotherapies
Psychotherapy and personality disorders	*Interface between psychiatry and neurology
Alcohol and substance abuse	Personality disorders
Ethical issues	*Schizophrenia and psychotic disorders
	Alcohol and substance abuse
Medical psychiatry	Ethical issues
Adjustment, mood and anxiety disorders	
Child and adolescent disorders	Medical psychiatry
4 case conferences	Adjustment, mood and anxiety disorders
	Child and adolescent disorders
	3 case conferences

TBL and articles/chapters about the psychiatric examination and clerkship policies. Sessions are conducted by the faculty who create them on our main campus, and by the clerkship director at the INOVA campus in northern Virginia.

TEAM FORMATION

During the academic year we have eight groups of students rotating through psychiatry. As there are 180 students in each class, each group will have 20–25 students on our main VCU campus, and about 5 students at the INOVA campus. Each team has 4–6 students; teams are formed the first day by asking students to indicate how well they feel they know the assignment for the day. Those who feel they know the material well are distributed equitably among the teams. We are careful to not assign any current or past "couples" to the same team, except at our INOVA campus where we have only one team per rotation.

READINESS ASSURANCE TESTS (RATS)

RATS range from 15 to 20 multiple-choice questions. Immediate Feedback-Assessment Technique (IF-AT) scratch-off forms are used for the GRAT.

TABLE 17.2
Objectives for Didactic Sessions Using TBL

TBL Session	Objectives
Orientation	• The student will be able to describe the components and workings of the psychiatry clerkship. • The student will be able to describe the components of the mental status exam and comprehensive psychiatric evaluation of a patient. • The student will be able to describe the principles of the biopsychosocial evaluation.
Psychopharmacology	• The student will be able to identify the indications and contraindications for medications commonly used in psychiatry. • The student will be able to identify the mechanisms, side effects, and common alternatives for medications commonly used in psychiatry.
The psychotherapies	• The student will be able to describe basic techniques used in psychodynamic/psychoanalytic therapy. • The student will be able to describe basic techniques used in behavioral/cognitive behavioral therapies. • The student will be able to describe basic techniques used in humanistic therapies.
Schizophrenia and related disorders	The student will understand the • basic pathophysiology of schizophrenia and other psychotic disorders. • pharmacological effects of antipsychotic medication. • epidemiology of psychotic disorders.
Interface between psychiatry and neurology	The student will begin to • discern psychiatric from neurological disorders when the patient's presenting symptoms relate to behavior. • appreciate the presentations of common neurologic disorders.

APPLICATION EXERCISES

Application exercises are created from one or two clinical cases, with several questions about each. Generally these are paper based, but one faculty member has used a PowerPoint presentation to inspire the deliberations. We adhere to the "simultaneous response" (Michaelsen & Knight, 2004) in the protocol using letter-coded laminated cards. Each team defends its rationale for its answers.

PEER EVALUATION

We require that each student provide qualitative feedback to each of his or her teammates in regard to preparation for class, contributions to the team's work, respect for one another, and flexibility during team disagreements. One hundred points are distributed within each team by each student, who also has the opportunity to make anonymous (to the peer) suggestions on how a teammate could be more helpful. Although most students choose to divide the points equitably, this is not required. We find that we are able to gather helpful information about professionalism with this evaluation, which can then be discussed with the student (see Figure 17.1).

OUTCOMES

We have used TBL in our didactic series for about one and one-half years. Students complete evaluations of the clerkship in two ways: on paper immediately after they complete the National Board of Medical Examiners subject exam in psychiatry (shelf exam), and on a Web site maintained by the school's curriculum office. Our first year of student evaluations was mixed in opinion, as others have found with an initial implementation. Specifically, many students do not like losing the lecture and being held accountable for the assigned readings. Some faculty missed not doing more lecture as well. We have continued to make changes to our exercises, including further consultation from Dr. Levine, and the internal medicine clerkship has begun to use TBL in its didactic series.

CONCLUSIONS/SUGGESTIONS

TBL is a viable alternative for medical school clerkship didactics for many reasons: enhances teamwork and the professional competencies of communication and respect for other professionals, increases the amount of reading that students will complete, and spares the faculty from having to repeat the same lecture every six weeks throughout the year. In our case, it would have helped our student response to TBL if the strategy had been adopted earlier by one or more other clerkships. We anxiously await later feedback from students and faculty across two or more clerkships to better understand the impact of the strategy and how we can continue to improve it.

FIGURE 17.1
Peer Evaluation

Below, please evaluate the contributions of each person in your group *except your-self*, by distributing 100 points among them. *Do not forget to include comments for each person.*

Team #:	Points Awarded:

1. Name:
   a. In what ways was your teammate *most* helpful to the team?
   b. In what ways could your teammate improve to be more effective?	

2. Name:
   a. In what ways was your teammate *most* helpful to the team?
   b. In what ways could your teammate improve to be more effective?	

3. Name:
   a. In what ways was your teammate *most* helpful to the team?
   b. In what ways could your teammate improve to be more effective?	

4. Name:
   a. In what ways was your teammate *most* helpful to the team?
   b. In what ways could your teammate improve to be more effective?	

5. Name:
   a. In what ways was your teammate *most* helpful to the team?
   b. In what ways could your teammate improve to be more effective?	

Your Name: **Total Points:**	100

REFERENCES

Armstrong, E. G. (1997). A hybrid model of problem-based learning. In D. Boud, & G. Feletti (Eds.), *The challenge of problem-based learning* (2nd ed., pp. 137–150). London: Kogan Page.

Arseneau, R., & Rodenburg, D. (1998). The developmental perspective—Cultivating ways of thinking. In D. D. Pratt (Ed.), *Five perspectives on teaching in adult and higher education* (pp. 105–149). Malabar, FL: Krieger.

Guild, P. B., & Garger, S. (1998). Curriculum: McCarthy's 4mat System. In P. B. Guild & S. Garger (Eds.), *Marching to different drummers* (2nd ed., pp. 50–59). Alexandria, VA: Association for Supervision and Curriculum Development.

Hoffman, K., & Headrick, L. (2006). Problem-based learning outcomes: Ten years of experience at the University of Missouri–Columbia School of Medicine. *Academic Medicine, 81,* 617–625.

Kaufman, D. (2003). ABC of learning and teaching in medicine—Applying educational theory in practice. *British Medical Journal, 326,* 213–216.

Kern, D. E., Thomas, P. A., Howard, D. M., & Bass, E. B. (1998). Step 4: Educational Strategies. In D. E. Kern, P. A. Thomas, D. M. Howard, & E. B. Bass (Eds.), *Curriculum development for medical education* (pp. 38–58). Baltimore: Johns Hopkins University Press.

Levine, R. E., O'Boyle, M., Haidet, P., Lynn, D. J., Stone, M. M., Wolf, D. V., et al. (2004). Transforming a clinical clerkship with team learning. *Teaching and Learning in Medicine, 16*(3), 270–275.

Michaelsen, L. K. (2004). Getting started with team learning. In L. K. Michaelsen, A. B. Knight, & L. D. Fink (Eds.), *Team-based learning: A transformative use of small groups in college teaching* (pp. 27–50). Sterling, VA: Stylus Publishing.

Michaelsen, L. K., & Knight, A. B. (2004). Creating effective assignments: A key component of team-based learning. In L. K. Michaelsen, A. B. Knight, & L. D. Fink (Eds.), *Team-based learning: A transformative use of small groups in college teaching* (pp. 51–57). Sterling, VA: Stylus.

Wass, V., van der Vleuten, C., Shatzer, J., & Jones, R. (2001). Assessment of clinical competence. *The Lancet, 357,* 945–949.

CHAPTER 18

Reinvigorating a Residency Program Through Team-Based Learning

The Experience of a Physical Medicine and Rehabilitation Program

Michael E. Petty and Kevin M. Means

A frequent complaint expressed by many residency program directors is that residents are not reading material assigned for seminars, conferences, and other didactic sessions. As a result, some residents appear to be uninterested, as faculty drone on with material they have presented numerous times through the years. Lack of motivation on the part of busy residents and lack of enthusiasm by some faculty members are symptoms of a deeper problem—a curriculum that employs teaching strategies that are relatively stagnant, with only content being updated as evidence of better clinical techniques are identified. This chapter presents team-based learning (TBL) as a teaching strategy, which changes the environment of didactic sessions in a manner that reinvigorates faculty, making them look forward to teaching again. The format requires residents to come to TBL sessions prepared, requiring faculty to ask more questions with greater depth, thus adding value to the didactic material by taking the residents outside the textbooks and research papers and into practical applications in the clinical setting.

Two perspectives of the implementation process are provided—that of the residency program director who chose to use the educational strategy, and that of the educational consultant who worked with faculty in coordinating the implementation. Both should be helpful to anyone considering TBL for their residency program. The chapter concludes with a road map to how you can proceed if you elect to implement TBL in your residency.

THE PROGRAM DIRECTOR'S PERSPECTIVE

TBL is a teaching strategy that has tremendous potential for graduate medical education in general, and for our physical medicine and rehabilitation residency program (PM&R), in particular. To understand why, a brief synopsis of our program and our experience with TBL to date is warranted.

RESIDENCY PROGRAM AND BACKGROUND

We are one of 80 PM&R residency programs in the United States. Founded in 1987, our four-year residency program is small to medium sized, averaging 14 residents (3 to 4 per year). Our PM&R faculty is relatively small in number, averaging 10 to 12 full-time faculty members over the past five years. Our residents and faculty are physically located in four different sites within Little Rock, Arkansas, corresponding to the locations of inpatient rehabilitation units of our affiliated hospitals. Residents and faculty converge in one central location for weekly educational sessions and clinical conferences.

Prior to the introduction of TBL, our residency program, like many others, relied heavily on traditional didactic lectures to highlight or communicate important medical knowledge that resident trainees must acquire. This didactic lecture series occurs in addition to hands-on clinical training and informal clinical teaching to which residents are exposed on a daily basis. The Residency Review Committee (RRC) for programs in PM&R, which oversees and establishes requirements for PM&R residency programs, mandates that programs have an organized series of lectures that address specific areas of medical knowledge in PM&R.

The overall didactic lecture program consists of multiple series of two to six lectures covering major topics (e.g., musculoskeletal disorders, electrodiagnosis, rehabilitation of persons with stroke, etc.). Each lecture series covers several subtopics. A PM&R faculty member coordinates each major lecture series and topic—usually a local content expert in that area—and each lecture in a series is presented by a PM&R faculty member or guest lecturer with notable expertise. The resident didactic lectures occur weekly and the entire didactic program is repeated every two years. These weekly lectures along with supplemental laboratory or practical hands-on sessions add up to about 100 lectures in the entire two-year cycle of lectures. Accordingly, updating and presenting about five lectures per year and coordinating two or three of the lecture series each year represents a significant teaching commitment for our PM&R faculty who also participate in numerous other academic activities in addition to maintaining full-time clinical practices. More than half of our faculty members are tenured associate or full professors with an average of 16 years of experience in the department.

CONDITIONS LEADING TO THE INTRODUCTION OF TBL

Several factors observed over the last several years contributed to our introducing TBL. These factors include (a) a perceived relative deterioration in our "environment of inquiry," (b) a decline in resident attendance at lectures, (c) a noticeable lack of reading on the part of residents, and (d) perceived faculty boredom with preparation and presentation of didactic lectures.

As program director I review evaluations of residents by faculty and evaluations of faculty by residents. I also conduct annual evaluative interviews for faculty and residents as well as exit interviews for departing faculty and graduating residents. Over the past four or five years, one of the most consistent comments made by (graduating) residents was that they felt that they were not asked many challenging questions by faculty and that the program could be improved by asking them more questions. Curiously, no residents raised this point until they were leaving the program. Consistent comments about residents by our faculty included observations that residents rarely asked questions, perhaps because faculty also felt that few residents read a sufficient amount of assigned readings.

Few residents were in the habit of reading or reviewing topics in advance of presented lectures. Questions from attendees during or after lectures were rare. Comments by several residents indicated that some faculty lectures were somewhat lacking in the area of delivery. I perceived that some faculty members might have been bored with presenting the same lectures and coordinating the same lecture series repeatedly. However, faculty members were reluctant to switch to a new lecture topic. It was difficult to find faculty volunteers for new lecture assignments that arose when a faculty member left the department, requiring a reassignment of that faculty member's lectures and series coordination responsibilities.

Too often, few residents attended didactic lectures and those who did attend were often unprepared and uninspired. Residents often joined faculty in a conspiracy of "don't ask and don't tell." Collectively, these circumstances were symptomatic of a relative decline in our environment of inquiry—something that had always been very strong for most of our program's existence. Several years ago, our program started a formal board examination preparation program for our residents. The program incorporates review of educational topics, review of multiple-choice examination questions, and participation in mock oral examinations. In recent years, resident interest in these board examination preparation sessions, as judged by attendance at and preparation for the sessions, paralleled that of the didactic lectures and began to wane.

Not surprisingly, we began to see a declining trend in overall resident performance on the annual American Academy of PM&R (AAPM&R) Self-Assessment Examination (SAE) and eventually on our overall performance on the American Board of Physical Medicine and Rehabilitation written and oral examinations. This was especially evident on the oral board examination that relies heavily on the integration of medical knowledge acquired during the residency and its application to patient care. In 2005, our RRC announced that effective in July 2006, the minimum required pass rate for residency programs on the board examination would be raised, making the declining trend in our board pass rate even more foreboding.

TBL INTRODUCTION AND IMPLEMENTATION

We decided to take preemptive action. Our university is fortunate to have an active Office of Educational Development (OED) that employs education specialists who are available to assist graduate medical education programs on our campus. In October 2005, shortly after reviewing our program's board performance statistics for

2005, I sought consultation advice from our OED. After a review of our program and academic situation, the outcome of this consultation was a suggestion that we consider introduction and implementation of TBL methodology into our educational program (see Figure 18.1 for a timetable outlining the actual implementation).

INTRODUCTION OF TBL TO THE PM&R FACULTY

The more I learned about TBL the more convinced I was that this is the ideal way to address and remedy the ominous educational issues affecting our residency program. I was also aware that implementing a significant change in teaching strategy among busy medical faculty members (especially experienced midcareer faculty) would likely be met with some degree of resistance. I did have one advantage. Because I serve as both residency program director and department chair, I already had the support and leadership for this endeavor from my chair.

I decided to take a gradual, multistage approach toward introducing TBL. First, I presented my observations and assessment of current trends and future possibilities for our educational program at a regularly scheduled faculty meeting, and invited open discussion. Next, I invited Petty (the OED consultant) to a specially called faculty meeting (December 2005) to present a basic description of the TBL process and to answer questions. The special meeting was an attempt to focus additional attention on this issue and to improve attendance at the faculty meeting, which is rarely 100 percent. The special meeting was well attended.

Coincidentally, our campus was planning to host a TBL workshop within a few weeks after our special faculty meeting (February 2006). I gently encouraged all PM&R faculty members to register for and attend this workshop. I was pleasantly surprised to see that, with the exception of one faculty member who was out of town for a family emergency, our entire faculty attended the workshop, as well as our chief

FIGURE 18.1
TBL Implementation Timeline

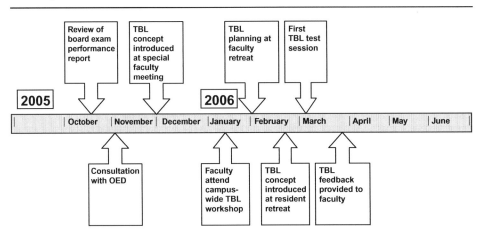

resident and our residency program coordinator. I noticed that our entire faculty seemed to enjoy the workshop and they actively and enthusiastically participated. Some faculty stayed after the workshop ended to ask questions of the presenter (Dean Parmelee). Feedback that I solicited from the faculty on the TBL workshop experience was positive.

To build on the enthusiasm stimulated by the TBL workshop, I committed a major part of our annual faculty retreat agenda (February 2006) to further training in TBL methods. This worked well as the retreat was two days after Parmelee's workshop. Led by Petty, the faculty worked on details related to TBL implementation planning, and development of related educational goals. Our faculty had clearly bought in to the TBL concept at that point. Many key matters were discussed and decisions made during this retreat session, such as which lecture series topics were or were not conducive to presentation using the TBL format, establishment and content of a reward system for the teams, and inclusion of and format for team and individual evaluations.

INTRODUCTION OF TBL TO PM&R RESIDENTS

The next step was to introduce the TBL concept to our PM&R residents. I did this by incorporating an educational session about TBL into part of the agenda of a scheduled annual resident retreat (also in February 2006). Because the chief resident also had attended the TBL workshop and informally had discussed this with some of the residents, it was easier to sell them on the TBL concept. I was able to announce the start of the first TBL session to the residents with about one month advance notice. During one of the non-TBL resident lectures, we divided the residents into their TBL teams. Excluding our first-year postgraduate (PGY-1) residents (who are not required to attend our didactic lectures), we had a total of nine residents and we decided to split them into two teams. Although one team would have an extra member, we assigned one of our residents (who already was planning to take an imminent extended maternity leave) to the group with the "extra" member. Also, we happened to have two international residents in our program, both of whom had already completed PM&R training abroad and were completing their second PM&R residency in order to practice in the United States. We intentionally assigned these two residents to different groups to avoid any group having a substantial advantage. The remaining residents were assigned to a group by lining them up according to the geographic east-to-west location of their birthplace and then they counted off. Odd numbers were assigned to Group #1 and even numbers to Group #2.

IMPLEMENTATION

To set an example as program director, I volunteered to lead off our transition to use the TBL method by being the first to incorporate TBL in an upcoming lecture series on PM&R research in February and March. Consistent with TBL methods, specific readings were assigned in advance of this lecture series. Lecture content was revised to build on the assigned readings and to focus on important topics that were underemphasized or difficult to cover in the readings.

Petty provided helpful assistance with developing the group Readiness Assurance Test (GRAT) and the individual Readiness Assurance Test (IRAT) questions. He also attended all sessions of the PM&R research lecture series and provided immediate feedback during the first TBL testing session. I also solicited feedback from the residents about the series and session. Their response was unanimously positive. I reported this feedback (as well as my own favorable impressions about the TBL session from a presenter/moderator's perspective) to the faculty at a faculty meeting (March 2006). Petty provided additional assistance to faculty who subsequently presented lectures using the TBL method.

TBL OUTCOMES

Currently, we are still midway in the process of transitioning most of the lectures in our two-year didactic lecture series to the TBL format. We plan to monitor key indicators that will allow us to assess the overall effect of TBL in our program. These indicators include our written and oral board examination scores and pass rate, scores on the AAPM&R SAE, lecture attendance statistics, and resident and faculty evaluation scores.

In addition to these important objective measurements, I have already made some preliminary and anecdotal observations that are more difficult to measure. Faculty and residents appear to be adjusting positively to this new TBL teaching and learning format. Since the implementation of TBL, residents not only are present and on time for lectures, they are also better prepared by reading the material in advance of the lecture sessions. Faculty now expect the residents to be prepared, and they accordingly are more likely to ask the residents thought-probing questions and are more likely to receive thoughtful answers. During the TBL sessions, it is exciting to see residents vigorously defend their answers to test questions based on knowledge of the literature and intelligently apply what they learned through reading and supplemental explanation in the TBL-based lectures. This type of active and productive faculty-resident exchange is extremely gratifying to faculty educators and resident learners alike.

While the longer-term objective effects of our TBL implementation await further investigation and appraisal, implementation of this promising teaching strategy already has produced positive and palpable systemic changes in our program. We feel that the TBL methodology and the attitudinal behavioral changes associated with implementing it have contributed to reinvigorating our program in a way that we anticipate will produce lasting benefits for years to come. To the extent that our program and experiences are typical of other programs—and we feel that at least some of them are—we believe that TBL is worth serious consideration as an alternative to the traditional lecture format.

THE CONSULTANT'S PERSPECTIVE:
FACULTY PREPARATION OF TBL SESSIONS

Residency faculty members employ a variety of techniques in the clinical teaching setting. Now, as they transitioned into the TBL format, their individual techniques and personalities came to the forefront. If a member was technologically savvy, he or she employed Web-based technologies to deliver content. A few continued to employ guest speakers with specialized knowledge to push residents beyond the textbook, while others extended the knowledge by using current research articles. All used personal experience as the cornerstone of highlighting points of emphasis.

These individual proclivities, along with the types of data used by their specific area of interest (radiographs, ambulatory aids, physical limitations, etc.), determined how IRAT/GRAT items were written and what forms of evidence were provided as background for these questions. Residency faculty members used clinical information to a much greater extent to develop these questions than had previously been observed in basic science or clerkship faculty's content questions. These required the use of diagnostic reasoning by residents, not only during the application phase, but also when taking the IRAT/GRAT.

With that stated, they also requested less assistance in preparing their TBL lessons. This was not a problem with the questions themselves, as faculty understood the "one-best-answer" format, but continuity across faculty in how they planned and taught the sessions became problematic. In one instance, a faculty member planned to have an IRAT with many more than 10 items. It really was to be a detailed test over content, not a quiz format. The "test" would have required a two-hour period just for the IRAT/GRAT phase. A simple solution was offered: provide the questions as study aids and choose 5 to 10 questions from that list for the IRAT. The faculty member liked the suggestion and had a very successful TBL session. Sufficient time became available to modify the scenarios during the appeals process and explore the impact of small variances in patient therapeutic presentation.

Another observation about residency faculty members is that they had difficulty promoting intergroup discussion. They were adept at allowing intragroup discussion during the GRAT and application phase, but when it came to discussion between groups over differences in rationale for specific choices, they became the "expert at the front of the room" too quickly. Different techniques were suggested and attempted to overcome this tendency (i.e., giving specific directions to groups, being at the back rather than at the front of the room, moving around the room), but it will require continued reinforcement to the faculty to instill this skill. The same tendency has been observed in faculty teaching clerkship students.

The application phase of TBL sessions followed a typical format seen in basic science or clerkship sessions. Clinical scenarios were presented and multiple-choice items offered, with all responses viable in certain clinical conditions. Groups discussed the scenarios, the possible choices, made one specific choice, and revealed them simultaneously. What differed at the resident level was that a much greater amount of visual information was used (radiographs, pictures, video, etc.). These provided information for the scenario that would have required extensive text to describe. This format also permitted faculty to detail personal experiences to highlight and differentiate when and why a particular wheelchair design would and would not be prescribed, why or why not a particular exercise routine would be employed, and how different gait problems presented. Much of this information was presented in study materials in preparation for the TBL session, but it further enhanced resident learning during the application phase.

One very positive modification that developed for use in the application phase was the addition of a prescription-writing exercise to culminate this phase. Following questions from residents, and detailed explanation and reflective questioning by faculty, the resident groups were asked to write a detailed prescription, providing the clinical basis for their specific recommendations. Both groups were required to explain their prescriptions to each other. Faculty and the opposite group's members offered critiques and recommendations. This exercise arose spontaneously from more than one faculty member and became a suggested practice for others (if appropriate for their subject area).

One thing must be emphasized: Don't constrain your faculty too much. While there are some basics of TBL that you want to coordinate across faculty for consistency, the faculty as individuals will be very creative in the session development process. While the content knowledge taught in basic science courses and clerkships place some constraint on faculty, residency education, with its emphasis on clinical knowledge, permits faculty more freedom to design their curriculum to support both their field and their teaching style.

OUTCOMES FROM STAKEHOLDERS' PERSPECTIVE

The PM&R residency program is in the early stages of this multiyear process. The program has employed TBL for only 10 months, and residents have not taken in-service exams that could be a measure of comparison for pre-TBL and post-TBL. Therefore, outcomes are the result of many conversations with Kevin Means, faculty, administrative staff, and residents. As previously attested, the departmental chair is pleased because he sees an enthusiastic faculty engaged with the TBL philosophy.

One or two faculty members have not yet become acquainted with TBL because of missing the retreat and not having taught to date, but those who have are enthusiastic about their experiences. They state that while the preparation time is significant, they do see better-prepared residents who are motivated to participate in the activities and willing to give opinions and ideas. Residents are attending sessions and they continue to be enthusiastic about the learning experiences they are receiving. They value the interaction with faculty, emphasizing the benefit of learning from the practical, clinically oriented faculty experiences they discuss each session.

One concern early on for the program was how to make the experience count for residents. In basic science and clerkship courses, grades are a strong motivator. Residents do not receive grades; therefore, another motivator was needed. To this end, a reward system involving textbook money was installed to encourage participation. As we progressed through the TBL sessions, it became apparent that, while the residents liked the reward system, the real motivators were team competition and interaction with the faculty. The tangible reward was least important of the three. Another residency program on campus that is initiating TBL is using conference funds in the program's final year of residency (rewarded for an 80% overall TBL grade) as the motivator.

A ROAD MAP FOR IMPLEMENTATION

Not everyone has the luxury of being both the residency program director and departmental chair, so I felt it beneficial to offer a road map, or checklist (if you prefer), to aid the planning process. As an educational development specialist, I would like to emphasize the need for quality control, at least at some level. Your time is very valuable, so comparing and contrasting faculty members' techniques will be a low priority, but some mechanism needs to be in place. I discovered idiosyncrasies that I did not anticipate.

The first step is to begin to understand TBL. If you have this book, you have already started that process. Table 18.1 offers direction beyond this. The key is gaining the support of decision makers. To comfortably do this, step 2 has to occur almost simultaneously with step 1 (some might argue before). You must ask the following questions:

What benefits can be anticipated for your program?
What is the purpose of considering the change?
Do you need to change?

Step 3 can be accomplished by you or someone experienced in TBL. It is critical, at this point, that the presenter understands the details of the TBL teaching strategy. I have found that a quick 15-minute synopsis has little impact and, in fact, is detrimental to your success; 30–60 minutes provides sufficient time for thorough presentation and discussion. You are attempting to build faculty enthusiasm at this point. Whenever possible, use change advocates among your faculty to help build faculty support. This was very easy for PM&R, as several faculty members quickly jumped on the bandwagon.

Once the faculty is interested, have a TBL workshop. Someone from the Team-Based Learning Collaborative (http://www.tlcollaborative.org/) can facilitate one.

TABLE 18.1
Road Map for Implementation of Team-Based Learning

1. Gain the interest of the course director/residency director/departmental chair
   a. TBL workshop (local or regional)
   b. One-on-one consult
2. Identify purpose for implementing TBL
   a. Raise test scores
   b. Raise level of interaction in class
   c. Raise interest level of faculty
3. Present basics of TBL to faculty
   a. Take sufficient time—does not work in 15 minutes
   b. Faculty meeting—one hour
4. Have the TBL workshop experience
   a. Bring in someone
   b. Do it yourself in a classroom setting
5. Have a defined session for beginning the development process
   a. Retreat
   b. Go to the clinician whenever possible
6. Have a defined review process for question writing
   a. Especially important with several faculty over an extended period of time
      i. Quality Control—Step 1
7. Have an observer critique the process of facilitating the session
   a. Faculty try to get too creative sometimes
      i. Quality Control—Step 2
8. Readjustment and feedback session
   a. Concerning what worked, went well, surprised, disappointed
      i. Quality Control—Step 3
9. Continue with faculty development

Bringing in an outside speaker adds to your credibility and also provides an opportunity to highlight your department by allowing you to invite others on campus to your department and learn about a new teaching strategy.

Step 4 involves a working session for your faculty. What worked well for PM&R was having a faculty retreat within one week of Dean Parmelee's workshop to begin finalizing the implementation plan. Enthusiasm was high after the workshop. We built on that enthusiasm at the retreat, and that enthusiasm has carried on throughout the process to date.

The steps from this point on focus on the quality control issues I mentioned earlier. Some faculty members want a tight review process for IRAT and application questions, while others do not. How "mandatory" you make step 6 is up to you, but it is a necessary step. At the least, someone needs to discuss the process with the faculty member responsible for the topic area and TBL session in advance to anticipate how he or she will conduct the session.

The next step is critical—someone needs to observe the TBL session to critique it. With a clerkship TBL session, the faculty member presents the session repetitively every one to three months, so consistency is simpler to obtain. PM&R TBL sessions are once every two years for a given topic area. Consistency is accomplished not by repetition of content but by repetition of processes across content areas.

The readjustment and feedback step is vital. This allows faculty, who are spread across five hospitals and two cities, to come together and discuss their experiences. To date this has only been accomplished informally with the PM&R faculty, and I am sure it will occur at the annual retreat, but sharing of perspectives along the way, especially early on, builds on that early enthusiasm and helps to identify weaknesses not visible to an external observer.

Finally, for a residency program, faculty development requires an extended time period because of the length of the program. A continuous quality improvement process will maintain faculty enthusiasm and continue to reinvigorate your faculty.

Contributors

CHERYL S. AL-MATEEN
Virginia Commonwealth University School of Medicine

Dr. Al-Mateen is Associate Professor of Psychiatry and the Director of the Clerkship in Psychiatry. She is a graduate of Howard University College of Medicine and completed residencies in both adult and child psychiatry. Her areas of scholarship include cultural competency and education and the effects of violence on children and adolescents.

JOHN D. BELL
Brigham Young University

Dr. Bell is the Associate Dean over Education in the College of Life Sciences at Brigham Young University in Provo, Utah. He graduated from the University of California, San Diego in 1987, with a Ph.D. in physiology and pharmacology. After completing three years of postdoctoral work in the Departments of Pharmacology and Biochemistry at the University of Virginia, he began his appointment at Brigham Young University in the Department of Zoology.

WILLIAM BRADSHAW
Brigham Young University

William S. Bradshaw is a Professor in the Department of Microbiology and Molecular Biology at Brigham Young University. His research interests include control of gene expression during embryonic development, molecular mechanisms of teratogenesis, and most recently, promoting the acquisition of analytical thinking skill by university students. He has also served the university as Associate Dean of the Honors Program.

MICHELE C. CLARK
University of Nevada at Las Vegas
School of Nursing

Michele C Clark, R.N., Ph.D., is an Associate Professor in the Psycho-social Nursing department at the University of Nevada at Las Vegas School of Nursing. Prior to joining UNLV School of Nursing in 2006, she was an Associate Professor in the community health department at the University of Texas Medical Branch in Galveston (UTMB). At UTMB School of Nursing she introduced Team-Based Learning (TBL) in 2005, and this teaching strategy has been successfully implemented in three required undergraduate nursing courses. She has also completed a small research study validating its efficacy with undergraduate students. Presently at UNLV School of Nursing, TBL has been introduced and used in the undergraduate community health course. Certain components of TBL (GRATS and application exercises) have also been implemented in an on-line doctoral course.

DAVID O. DEFOUW
New Jersey Medical School

Dr. DeFouw is Vice Chair and Director of educational programs in the Department of Cell Biology and Molecular Medicine. He serves as the course director for the first-year medical courses Human Anatomy and Development and Integrated Structure and Function. In addition, he participates in several graduate courses that cover various aspects of cell biology. His research interests have focused on endothelial cell biology with an emphasis on differentiation of endothelial permselectivity during normal angiogenesis.

DOROTHY BALDWIN ENGLE
Xavier University

Dr. Engle is an Associate Professor in the Biology Department of Xavier University in Cincinnati, OH. She is a graduate of Carnegie-Mellon University and completed post-doctoral training at University of Medicine and Dentistry of New Jersey Robert Wood Johnson Medical School and at the University of Cincinnati College of Medicine. A past recipient of awards for excellence in teaching, she has instituted Team-Based Learning into the genetics courses in the premedical curriculum at Xavier University. She presented at the TBL Workshop in 2005 and contributed an article for an on-campus faculty development publication. She has also spread the TBL gospel as a mentor for several graduate students in the University of Cincinnati's Preparing Future Faculty Program.

TERESA A. GARRETT
Vassar College

Dr. Garrett is currently an Assistant Professor of Chemistry at Vassar College. Prior to joining the faculty of Vassar, she was an Assistant Research Professor in the Department of Biochemistry at Duke University Medical Center. While at Duke, she began introducing Team-Based Learning in her teaching of medical and undergraduate students. She plans to continue using Team-Based Learning in her classes at Vassar College.

PAUL HAIDET
The Michael E. DeBakey Veterans Affairs Medical Center
and Baylor College of Medicine

Dr. Haidet is a clinician educator and researcher at the Houston Center for Quality of Care and Utilization Studies, a Department of Veterans Affairs Center of Excellence in Health Services Research. He has performed work funded by the U.S. Department of Education to implement, evaluate, and disseminate Team-Based Learning in medical education. He is currently the Research Director for the Team-Based Learning Collaborative, a nonprofit organization devoted to supporting educators interested in TBL. Dr. Haidet has conducted over 20 TBL workshops at medical schools across the United States, and has published 10 articles about the method in the medical literature.

HERBERT FREDERICK JANSSEN
Texas Tech University Health Sciences Center

Dr. Janssen is a Professor and Associate Chair for Research in the Department of Orthopaedic Surgery and Rehabilitation at Texas Tech University Health Sciences Center in Lubbock, Texas. He has a joint appointment in the Department of Cell Physiology and Molecular Biophysics. He teaches residents, undergraduate, graduate, and medical students. Dr. Janssen has served as a faculty advisor on graduate committees in education, engineering, and the medical sciences. He has published numerous articles, book chapters, and two books. He has conducted workshops promoting active learning and critical thinking in the medical sciences.

KARLA A. KUBITZ
Towson University

Dr. Kubitz received her Ph.D. in Exercise Science from Arizona State University. She is currently an Associate Professor in the Department of Kinesiology at Towson University in Towson, Maryland and has been successfully using Team-Based Learning for several years in her sport and exercise psychology classes.

RUTH E. LEVINE
University of Texas Medical Branch

Dr. Levine is the Clarence Ross Miller Professor of Psychiatry in the Department of Psychiatry and Behavioral Sciences at the University of Texas Medical Branch (UTMB), where she has served on the faculty for 16 years. Since 1995 she has been Director of Medical Student Education for the department. She is also the inaugural director of UTMB's Academy of Master Teachers, established in 2006. She received her medical degree from UTMB and completed her residency in general psychiatry at the Boston University School of Medicine. Dr. Levine has established Team-Based Learning courses in undergraduate, graduate, and postgraduate medical settings, and has provided workshops and consultative services to numerous faculty in the United States and Canada. She has also authored a number of publications outlining her experiences with Team-Based Learning.

KATHRYN K. McMAHON
Texas Tech University Health Sciences Center

Dr. McMahon is the Associate Professor in the Department of Pharmacology and Neuroscience at Texas Tech University Health Sciences Center in Lubbock. She is a graduate of North Dakota State University and received postdoctoral training at Rutgers Medical School and at Chicago Medical School. At the Texas Tech School of Medicine, she introduced Team-Based Learning (TBL) into the first- and second-year curricula as an alternative and supplement to lecture teaching to enhance medical students' integration of information via *active learning*. She has conducted TBL workshops at national medical education and scientific meetings in the past five years throughout the United States, and is author of numerous publications.

KEVIN M. MEANS
College of Medicine, University of Arkansas for Medical Sciences

Dr. Means is Professor, Chair, and Residency Program Director of the Department of Physical Medicine & Rehabilitation in the College of Medicine at the University of Arkansas for Medical Sciences. He holds clinical appointments at University Hospital of Arkansas, the Central Arkansas Veterans Healthcare System, and at Baptist Health Rehabilitation Institute (BHRI), where he is also the Medical Director. He is a Board-certified physician in the specialty of physical medicine and rehabilitation. Dr. Means conducts research in the area of falls prevention in the elderly and has published numerous papers in peer-reviewed journals. Dr. Means is a graduate of Howard University College of Medicine. He completed residency training at the Rehabilitation Institute of Chicago/Northwestern University. He completed postgraduate work in health services research with the Scholars Program of the Center for Outcomes Research and Effectiveness, University of Arkansas for Medical Sciences, and additional postresidency training at On the Job/Off Campus Program in Clinical Research Design and Statistical Analysis, School of Public Health, University of Michigan. Dr. Means is the first Residency Program Director in the United States to institute Team-Based Learning (TBL) as a major teaching methodology in the residency curriculum. He has given several presentations on the introduction and use of TBL in graduate medical education.

LARRY K. MICHAELSEN
Central Missouri State University

Larry K. Michaelsen (Ph.D. in Organizational Psychology from The University of Michigan) is David Ross Boyd Professor Emeritus at the University of Oklahoma, Professor of Management at Central Missouri State University, a Carnegie Scholar, a Fulbright Senior Scholar, and former editor of the *Journal of Management Education*. He is active in faculty and staff development activities and has conducted over 300 workshops on various aspects of teaching effectively with small groups in a wide variety of university and corporate settings. Dr. Michaelsen has also received numerous college, university, and national awards for his outstanding teaching and for his pioneering work in two areas. One is the development of Team-Based Learning. The other is an Integrative Business Experience (IBE) program that links student learning in multiple core business courses to their experience in creating and operating an actual start-up business whose profits are used to fund hands-on community service work.

GARY M. ONADY
Wright State University Boonshoft School of Medicine

Dr. Onady is Associate Professor of Pediatrics and Internal Medicine at the Boonshoft School of Medicine of Wright State University in Dayton, Ohio. He currently directs the Dayton Adult Cystic Fibrosis Program; he served previously as the Director of the Combined Internal Medicine-Pediatrics residency program at Wright State University. He earned a graduate degree in chemistry at the City University of New

York, with postgraduate pharmacology training at Case Western Reserve University, and subsequently graduated from Wright State University School of Medicine. He completed residency training at Cleveland Metro General Hospital. Additionally, he is a professional jazz trumpeter and flugelhornist currently performing with the Eddie Brookshire Quintet.

DEAN X. PARMELEE
Wright State University Boonshoft School of Medicine

Dr. Parmelee is the Associate Dean for Academic Affairs at the Boonshoft School of Medicine of Wright State University in Dayton, Ohio, and Professor of Psychiatry and Pediatrics. Prior to joining Wright State in 2001, he was Chairman of the Division of Child & Adolescent Psychiatry and Professor of Psychiatry & Pediatrics at the Virginia Commonwealth University Medical College of Virginia. He is a graduate of the University of Rochester School of Medicine and completed his residencies at the Massachusetts General and McLean Hospitals of the Harvard Medical School. At the Boonshoft School of Medicine, he has pioneered Team-Based Learning (TBL) throughout its curriculum as an alternative and supplement to lecture teaching and to enhance medical student *active learning* and *teamwork.* He has conducted over 25 workshops for medical school faculty in the past two years throughout the United States and Singapore, is author of numerous publications, including two texts, and is the current co-editor of *Team-Based Learning in Health Professions Education.*

JOHN W. PELLEY
Texas Tech University Health Sciences Center School of Medicine

Dr. Pelley has been an Associate Professor of Biochemistry for the past 35 years at the Texas Tech University Health Sciences Center School of Medicine in Lubbock, Texas. During that time he has served as Admissions Dean, Associate Dean for Academic Affairs, and Interim Department Chairman. He has authored several books in medical biochemistry as well as a book on academic achievement for medical students. He has presented over 100 workshops and lectures to both medical students and faculty for the past 10 years.

MICHAEL E. PETTY
Rush University
Center for Medical Education and Research

Dr. Petty recently joined the Office of Medical Student Programs at Rush University in their new Center for Medical Education and Research. He holds Master of Science degrees in both Biology and Management from Purdue University, as well as a Ph.D.

in Curriculum and Instruction, Science Education, from Indiana University. Prior to moving to Rush he was in the Office of Educational Development at the University of Arkansas for Medical Sciences (UAMS) with a focus on both UME curricular development and GME accreditation. Dr. Petty was instrumental in the implementation of Team-Based Learning (TBL) at UAMS, particularly within the Physical Medicine and Rehabilitation residency program, Obstetrics and Gynecology clerkship, and its use in the Physiology curriculum in conjunction with their simulation experience in Cardiovascular and Respiratory blocks. He is currently working to implement TBL into faculty development curriculum at Rush.

ROBERT J. PHILPOT, JR.
South University

Dr. Philpot is an Associate Professor and Chairman of the Department of Physician Assistant Studies at South University in Savannah, Georgia. Prior to joining South University in 2006, he served on the faculty of the University of Florida College of Medicine Physician Assistant Program. He is a graduate of the Emory University of College of Medicine Physician Assistant Program and completed his Ph.D. at the University of Florida College of Education. He currently serves as the Executive Director for the Team-Based Learning (TBL) Collaborative, a nonprofit organization of educators whose purpose is to support other faculty, to share teaching resources, and to promote evaluation and research on Team-Based Learning. At the University of Florida College of Medicine and at South University he developed a number of innovative ways to integrate TBL into the physician assistant curriculum as a means of building critical thinking and problem-solving skills. He continues to conduct TBL workshops for faculty across the United States.

VIRGINIA SCHNEIDER
University of Texas M.D. Anderson Cancer Center

Virginia Schneider, PA-C, is a physician assistant with the University of Texas M.D. Anderson Cancer Center. Prior to joining M.D. Anderson, she was a founding member and later the Executive Director of the Team-Based Learning Collaborative, a national organization of TBL educators in health sciences education. An Assistant Professor of Pediatrics and Family and Community Medicine at Baylor College of Medicine, and an Adjunct Professor in the College of Pharmacy at the University of Houston, she used TBL extensively with medical, physician assistant, nursing, pharmacy, and graduate science students. Through expertise gathered as a co-investigator on the initial FIPSE grant adapting TBL in medical education, she mentored faculty and has given workshops and presentations on TBL nationally and internationally.

ROBERT C. SCHUTT, JR.
Texas Tech University Health Sciences Center

Dr. Schutt is the Chairman of the Department of Orthopaedic Surgery and Rehabilitation at Texas Tech University School of Medicine in Lubbock, Texas. Prior to joining Texas Tech in 2003, he was in private practice in Colorado Springs, Colorado.He is a graduate of Texas Tech University School of Medicine and completed his surgical internship at The University of Oklahoma and Orthopaedic Surgery residency at The University of Colorado. His clinical practice is currently limited to Pediatric Orthopaedics. At Texas Tech School of Medicine, he has developed curriculum and actively participates in the teaching of orthopaedic residents and medical students. He is the author of numerous publications and presentations related to Team-Based Learning.

NICHOLAS P. SKEEN
Texas Tech University Health Sciences Center

Nicholas Skeen holds a Bachelors degree in Microbiology from Texas Tech University and is currently pursuing an MBA. He is a Research Associate at Texas Tech University Health Sciences Center where he conducts research and manages the activities of the Ershel Franklin Memorial Tissue Bank. He has helped develop activity learning modules for students in undergraduate and medical education. Mr. Skeen has also designed and presented the results of several research projects dealing with critical thinking in the medical sciences.

MICHAEL SWEET
University of Texas at Austin

Michael Sweet, currently a Ph.D. candidate at the University of Texas at Austin, is an instructional consultant for the Division of Instructional Innovation and Assessment (DIIA) at the University of Texas at Austin. He has been a college-level instructional consultant for more than a decade, helping teachers of all ranks in all disciplines to activate their classrooms, primarily with TBL. Michael has published and presented widely on collaborative learning methods in higher education, and recently guest-edited a special issue of *Educational Psychology Review* on the topic.

NAGASWAMI S. VASAN
New Jersey Medical School

Dr. Vasan is an Associate Professor in the Department of Cell Biology and Molecular Medicine at New Jersey Medical School. He has been teaching anatomy for 33 years, and has served as course director for the medical anatomy program for 13 years. He has successfully implemented TBL in medical and graduate anatomy programs. In collaboration with other colleagues, he conducts TBL workshops or discussions at the AAMC annual meeting and other venues, and has published work on his TBL experiences. He has also been a Harvard Macy Scholar and the first one in that program to develop TBL as his project.

Index

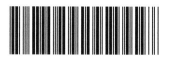